Gastric Sleeve Cookbook 2022

Simple, Healthy and Most Delicious Recipes after Weight Loss Surgery

TABLE OF CONTENTS

Introduction

Gastric detour scientific manner is certifiably now not an otherworldly system for buying more in shape. It's something but a "convenient solution." You may be powerful on the off threat that you alternate the way in that you consume for an extremely good the rest. This handbook gives a diagram of what you need to know.

The medical procedure works in two distinct approaches:

To begin with, the medical manner diminishes the sum your belly will hold from a thousand ml (4 cups) to 30 ml (2 Tbsp). A thousand ml is ready the size of a football, and 30 ml is set the dimensions of a hardboiled egg. This decreases the measure of nourishment you can consume at someone time (which is called confinement). You will sense complete inside the wake of eating tremendously little suppers and will, in this manner, eat less by using and big.

Second, nourishment sidesteps some part of your digestive tract, which lessens what amount is retained from the sustenance's you eat (which is called malabsorption). A few human beings cannot undergo sugary and greasy sustenance's after the clinical method in view of the new changes, which inspires them to live far away from those fatty nourishments.

Joined with well-known exercise, the gastric detour diet will permit you to get thinner and keep it off. Most patients will lose up to 50-70% in their abundance bodyweight inside years. In any case, on the off chance which you do not pursue the healthful policies, you can create medical troubles and may even restore the weight. Other than developing notable consuming and exercising propensities, non-stop advising could make new inclinations towards sustenance and preserve terrible behavior styles from returning. The data gave in this e-book will allow you to develop new eating examples and guarantee a strong weight loss.

Gastric Sleeve Breakfast Recipes

Blackberry Almond Butter Sandwich

Prep Time: 30mins Cook Time: 0mins , SERVES: 1

INGREDIENTS
- ¼ - cup blackberries
- 1 - teaspoon chia seeds
- 2 - slices 100-percent whole wheat bread, lightly toasted
- 2 - tablespoons natural almond butter

Instructions:
- In a bowl, pound blackberries softly with a fork. Mix in chia seeds.
- Discretionary: Cover and refrigerate blackberry-chia blend for as long as 4 days for a thick, jamlike consistency.
- Collect sandwich with blackberry blend more than one cut of bread and almond margarine over another cut.

NUTRITION PER SERVING
Calories 445, Fat 19g, Carbs 52g, Sugar 11g, Protein 19g.

Blackberry Vanilla French Toast

Prep Time: 10mins Cook Time: 50mins , SERVES: 2

INGREDIENTS

- 4 - eggs, beaten
- ½ - teaspoon vanilla extract
- Salt
- 4 - slices whole wheat bread
- 1 - cup fresh blackberries
- 20 - pecan halves, chopped
- 2 - teaspoons maple syrup

Instructions:

- In a shallow dish, mix eggs, vanilla, and a gap of salt altogether. Absorb cuts of bread egg blend, every cut in flip, till all of the egg is retained.
- In a big, nonstick skillet protected with cooking bathe over medium warm temperature, consist of the two drenched bread cuts and cook dinner until underside is awesome darker around 3 minutes. Flip and prepare dinner until fantastic dark-colored and quite firm, around 3 minutes extra.
- Rehash with the staying bread cuts and the rest of the egg combination.
- Top with blackberries, walnuts, and maple syrup.

NUTRITION PER SERVING:

Calories 434, Fat 17g, Carbs 49g, Sugar 14g, Protein 22g.

Chocolate-Peanut Butter French Toast

INGREDIENTS

- 1/3 - cup liquid egg whites
- 2 - teaspoons unsweetened cocoa powder
- ½ - teaspoon vanilla extract
- Salt
- 2 - slices whole-grain bread
- 1 - tablespoon peanut butter
- 2/3 - cup fresh raspberries

Instructions:

- In a shallow dish or bowl, whisk collectively egg whites, cocoa powder, vanilla, and a touch of salt. Absorb bread egg blend, each reduce in flip, until all the egg is ingested.
- In an giant, nonstick skillet blanketed with cooking splash over medium warmth, consist of bread cuts and cook dinner till underside is dim brilliant darker, round 3mints. Flip and cook until terrific darkish coloured and marginally firm, round 3mints greater.
- Spread nutty unfold on French toast. Top with raspberries.

NUTRITION PER SERVING: *Calories 404, Carbs 52g, Protein 21g*

Watermelon Quinoa Parfait

Prep Time: 15mins Cook Time: 20mins , SERVES: 1

INGREDIENTS
- 1 - cup watermelon, cut into bite-sized pieces
- ½ - cup cooked quinoa
- 1 - tablespoon fresh mint, chopped
- ½ - cup plain 2-percent-fat Greek yogurt
- 20 - almonds, chopped

Instructions:
- In a bowl, mix together watermelon, quinoa, and mint.
- In a container or bowl, layer watermelon-quinoa blend with yogurt. Top with almonds.

NUTRITION PER SERVING:
Calories 411, Fat 17g, Carbs 42g, sugar 17g, Protein 25g.

Apple and Goat Cheese Sandwich

Prep Time: 5mins Cook Time: 5mins , SERVES: 1

INGREDIENTS
- 2 - slices 100-percent whole-wheat bread, toasted
- 1 - ounce goat cheese, at room temperature
- 1 - tablespoons natural peanut butter
- ½ - medium apple, cored and thinly sliced, divided
- ¼ - teaspoon cinnamon

Instructions:
- Spread 1 bit of toast with goat cheddar and the other with nutty spread. Make a sandwich with a large portion of the apple cuts sprinkled with cinnamon.
- Present with residual apple cuts.

NUTRITION PER SERVING: *Calories 408, Fat 17g, Carbs 49g, Sugar 15g, Protein 17g.*

Carrot Cake Oatmeal

Prep Time: 5mins Cook Time: 50mins , SERVES: 1

INGREDIENTS
- ½ - cup unsweetened almond milk
- 1 - small carrot, peeled and finely grated
- 1/3 - cup rolled oats
- 1 -tablespoon raisins
- 1 - teaspoon honey
- ¼ - teaspoon vanilla extract
- 1 - pinch cinnamon
- 1 - pinch salt
- 1 ½ - tablespoons peanut butter
- 1/3 - cup lowfat cottage cheese

Instructions:
- In a bit pot, be part of almond milk, half cup water, carrot, oats, raisins, nectar, vanilla, cinnamon, and salt. Heat to the factor of boiling, at that point, reduce to stew and cook, mixing sporadically, until thick and oats are stout, 5 to 7mints.
- Blend inside the nutty unfold and take out from the heat.
- Top cereal with curds and extra cinnamon.

NUTRITION PER SERVING:
Calories 423, Fat 17g, Carbs 51g, Protein 21g.

Coconut Cranberry Protein Bars

Prep Time: 20mins Cook Time: 0mins , SERVES: 1

Ingredients

- ¼ - cup unsweetened shredded coconut flakes
- ¼ - cup organic dried cranberries
- ¼ - cup almond butter
- 2 - tbsp almond meal
- 2 - tbsp flax meal
- 3 - tbsp coconut oil
- 1 - tbsp raw honey
- 2 - eggs
- 6 - scoops SFH Coconut Fuel Protein
- Dash Himalayan sea salt
- Optional: 1/4 Organic dark chocolate chunks/Enjoy Life's Chocolate Chips

Instructions:

- Preheat stove to 350
- Come to all fixings in a bowl and blend until a batter-like consistency
- Line an 8x8 preparing dish with material paper
- Take off batter into a level and even square
- Prepare for 15 to 20mints or until somewhat solidified
- Let cool and cut into squares

NUTRITION PER SERVING: *Calories 214, Fat 12.2g, Carb 8.2g, Sugars 3.1g, Protein 20g*

Egg White Oatmeal With Strawberries and Peanut Butter

Prep Time: 5mins Cook Time: 10mins , SERVES: 1

INGREDIENTS

- ½ - cup rolled oats
- ½ - cup unsweetened almond milk
- 6 - large fresh (or frozen, thawed) strawberries, cored and chopped
- 2 - teaspoons honey
- ½ - teaspoon vanilla extract
- 1 - pinch salt
- 1/3 - cup liquid egg whites
- 1 - tablespoon peanut butter

Instructions:

- In a little pot, heat oats, 1/2 cup almond milk, 1/3 cup water, strawberries, nectar, vanilla, and salt. Heat to the point of boiling, at that point decrease to stew and cook, blending once in a while, until the blend is thick and oats are full, 5 to 7mints. Expel from warm.
- In a bowl, whisk egg whites until somewhat bubbly. Add cooked cereal to egg whites a spoonful at once, rushing between every option, until oats are completely joined.
- Pour blend once more into the pot and cook over low heat, mixing always, until oats are thick, 2 to 3mints. Be mindful so as not to turn the warmth excessively high so eggs don't scramble.
- Top cereal with nutty spread.

NUTRITION PER SERVING: *Calories 412, Carbs 51g, Sugar 17g, Protein 20g.*

Low Carb Cottage Cheese Pancakes

Prep Time: 5mints Cook Time: 5mints , Servings: 1

Ingredients

- ½ - cup low-fat cottage cheese
- ¼ - cup oats
- ⅓ - cup egg Whites (2 egg whites)
- 1 - tsp. vanilla extract
- 1 - tbsp. Stevia in the raw

Instructions

- Pour curds and egg whites into the blender first, at that point include oats, vanilla concentrate, and a little stevia.
- Mix to a smooth consistency.
- Put a container with a bit of cooking shower on medium warmth and fry every hotcake until brilliant on the two sides.
- Present with berries, without sugar jam or nutty spread.

NUTRITION PER SERVING:

Calories 205, Fat 1.5g, Carb 19g, Sugar 5.5g, Protein 24.5g

Thai Chopped Chicken Salad with Peanut Vinaigrette

Prep Time: 20mins Cook Time: 0mins , SERVES: 2

Ingredients

Salad:

- 2 - heads Romaine Lettuce
- 2 - Bell Peppers, any color, thinly sliced
- 1 - Mango, sliced
- 1 - cup Shredded Carrots
- ½ - cup Roasted and Unsalted Peanuts
- 2 - cups Cooked Shredded Chicken

Spicy Peanut Dressing:

- 4 - Tbsp Thai Peanut Sauce
- 2 - Tbsp Olive Oil
- 2 - tsp Honey
- 2 - tsp Rice Vinegar
- 2 - tsp Lime Juice

Instructions

- Finely hack the lettuce and cut peppers and mango into slight strips. Toss lettuce, peppers, mango, carrots, peanuts, and chicken.
- Make the dressing by whisking together shelled nut sauce, oil, nectar, vinegar and lime juice. Taste and change in accordance with your inclination, including more nectar on the off chance that you'd like it all the more sweet or lime juice on the off chance that you'd like it progressively tart.
- Just before serving, add a large portion of the dressing to the plate of mixed greens and hurl well. Serve a plate of mixed greens with staying half of dressing as an afterthought and add to your inclination.

NUTRITION PER SERVING: *Calories: 351, Carb: 36g, Protein: 19g, Fat: 18g, Sugar: 23g*

California Steak Salad with Chimichurri Dressing

Prep Time: 5mins Cook Time: 20mins Total Time: 25mins
Serving Size: 2

Ingredients

- 1.25lb flank steak
- 1 - tablespoon olive oil
- Salt & pepper to season
- 8 oz. fresh arugula
- 1 - red onion, sliced into 1" rings
- 1lb - asparagus, trimmed
- 1 - pint of assorted cherry tomatoes, halved
- 1 - avocado, sliced
- **Chimichurri Dressing:**
- 1 - garlic clove
- 1 - cup fresh cilantro
- 2 - tablespoon red wine vinegar
- 1 - tablespoon lime juice
- 3 - tablespoons olive oil
- ¼ - teaspoon smoked paprika
- ½ - teaspoon red pepper flakes
- Salt & pepper to taste

Instructions

- Preheat barbeque to medium-excessive heat.
- Season asparagus and onion jewelry with olive oil and salt.
- Set asparagus and onion earrings at the fish fry. Barbecue the asparagus for 5mints. Flame broil the onion rings for 5mints on every facet until scorch imprints show up. Take out and mounted a at ease spot.
- Add 1 tablespoon of olive to flank steak, rub into every element. Season the two aspects with salt and pepper.
- Spot flank steak at the barbeque. Flame broil every factor for 3 to 5mints. Let relaxation for 5mints earlier than reducing.
- While the steak is resting add the accompanying to a chunk sustenance processor: a garlic clove, new cilantro, purple wine vinegar, olive oil, lime juice, smoked paprika, red pepper quantities, salt, and pepper. Mix till clean and resembles a dressing.
- Collect the serving of blended veggies, embody crisp arugula, flame-broiled red onion cuts, asparagus, cherry tomatoes, cut avocado, and reduce flank steak to a

big serving platter. Present with Chimichurri Dressing as an afterthought! Topping with a lime.

NUTRITION PER SERVING: *Calories: 452, Sugar: 6g, Fat: 32g, Carb: 16g, Protein: 36g*

Berry Cheesecake Overnight Oats

Prep Time: 5mins Cook Time: 5mins , SERVES: 1

INGREDIENTS:
- ½ - cup fresh (or frozen, thawed) blueberries
- 1 - teaspoon honey
- ½ - teaspoon vanilla extract
- ½ - cup rolled oats
- ½ - cup lowfat cottage cheese
- ½ - cup unsweetened almond milk
- 12 - almonds, chopped

Instructions:
- In a bowl or container, consolidate berries, nectar, and vanilla and squash with a fork. Include oats, curds, and almond milk, and mix to join. (The blend will be thick and might appear to be dry, yet the oats will relax as they sit.)
- Refrigerate in any event 6hrs.
- Serve cold, sprinkled with almonds.

NUTRITION PER SERVING: *Calories 406, Carbs 48g, Sugar 11g, Protein 24g.*

Pumpkin Protein Pancakes

Prep Time: 10mins Cook Time: 10mins , SERVES: 2

INGREDIENTS

- 2 - large eggs
- ¾ - cup plain 2-percent-fat Greek yogurt
- ½ - cup canned pumpkin
- 1 ½ - tablespoons maple syrup, divided
- ½ - teaspoon vanilla extract
- ½ - cup whole wheat flour
- ¼ - cup rolled oats
- 1 - teaspoon baking powder
- 1 - pinch salt
- ¼ - teaspoon pumpkin pie spice
- 20 - pecan halves, chopped

Instructions:

- In a bowl, beat eggs. Blend in yogurt, pumpkin, 1 tbsp maple syrup, and vanilla.
- In another bowl, blend together flour, oats, preparing powder, salt, and pumpkin pie flavor.
- Add dry fixings to wet and blend to consolidate.
- In an enormous nonstick skillet covered with cooking splash over medium-low heat, drop a loading ⅓ cup hitter for every flapjack. Cook until underside is darker and air pockets structure on top, around 3 minutes. Flip and cook around 3mints more. Rehash with residual hitter.
- Top with walnut parts and the rest of the maple syrup.
- Cool extra hotcakes before putting away in an impenetrable holder in the ice chest as long as 3 days, or store remaining hitter in a sealed shut compartment in the ice chest as long as 4 days.

NUTRITION PER SERVING: *Calories 415, Carbs 49g, Sugar 15g, Protein 22g.*

AVOCADO TOAST WITH COTTAGE CHEESE & TOMATOES

Prep Time: 5mins Cook Time: 5mins , SERVES: 4

INGREDIENTS

- 8 - slices hearty whole grain bread
- 2 - cups cottage cheese low fat
- 1 - ripe California avocado sliced

- 1 - tomato sliced
- Salt and freshly cracked pepper to taste

INSTRUCTIONS

- Lay bread cuts out on an enormous cutting board and tops everyone with ¼ cup of curds. Sprinkle with salt and pepper.
- Top curds with avocado and tomato cut at that point season with another spot of salt and pepper.
- Cut bread cuts down the middle and serve.

NUTRITION PER SERVING:

Calories 440, Fat 11.9g, Carb 63.5g Protein 25g

Savory Parmesan Oatmeal

Prep Time: 10mins Cook Time: 35mins , SERVES: 1

INGREDIENTS

- 1 - cup unsweetened almond milk
- 2/3 - cup rolled oats
- ½ - cup kale leaves, chopped
- ½ - cup broccoli florets, chopped
- Salt
- Pepper
- 1 - ounce Parmesan, grated

Instructions:

- In a touch pot, warm temperature almond milk, 1/3 cup water, oats, kale, and broccoli. Season with salt and pepper.
- Heat to the point of boiling, at that thing, decrease to stew and prepare dinner, blending at instances, till oats are whole, kale is withered, and broccoli is cooked although pretty company, 5 to 7mints.
- Top with Parmesan.

NUTRITION PER SERVING:
Calories 392, Carbs 45g, Sugar 3g, Protein 21g.

Strawberry Cheesecake Chia Seed Pudding

Prep time: 10mints Additional time: 1day , SERVING: 1

Ingredients

- ¼ - cup cottage cheese
- 1 - tbs greek yogurt
- 1 - cup chopped strawberries, divided
- ½ - cup almond milk
- 1/8 - tsp vanilla
- 2 - tsp raw sugar
- 2 - Tbs chia seeds

Instructions

- In a blender, join the curds, greek yogurt, 1/2 cup strawberries, almond milk, vanilla, and crude sugar and mix, mix, mix until the blend is totally smooth and lovably pink. You may need to scratch down with a spatula once in the middle.
- Fill a lidded holder and include the chia seeds, mixing admirably. Let sit medium-term (at any rate 24 hours, the more it sets, the thicker it gets!) in the cooler.
- The following day when you are prepared to eat it, blend it again to appropriate the seeds equitably and present with the staying 1/2 cup slashed strawberries. Yum

NUTRITION PER SERVING:*CALORIES: 245 TOTAL FAT: 8g*

Gastric Sleeve Lunch Recipes

BUFFALO CHICKEN CUPS

Prep: 5mins, Cook: 40mins Total: 45mins, Serving: 24

INGREDIENTS:

- 2 to 3 boneless, skinless chicken breasts
- 2 - Tbsp. olive oil
- ½ - tsp. smoked paprika
- ½ - tsp. chili powder
- 24 - wonton wrappers
- 1 - Tbsp. butter, melted
- ½ - cup cayenne hot sauce
- ½ - cup blue cheese crumbles
- 3 - scallions, sliced thinly

Instructions:

- Preheat broiler to 350F degrees.
- Brush chicken bosoms with olive oil, and after that sprinkle equitably with the smoked paprika and bean stew powder. Spot in a heating dish and cook for 20-30 minutes, or until the middle is never again pink and the juices run clear. Expel chicken and let cool, at that point shred.
- In the interim, fit a wonton wrapper into every one of 24 little preparing cups, squeezing the wrappers cautiously yet solidly into sides of cups. (Be mindful so as to keep the sides of every wonton wrapper open; else, you won't have the option to fill them!) Bake for 5mints or until daintily seared. Keep wontons in prepared cups.
- In a medium-sized bowl, mix together the dissolved spread and hot sauce. Include the chicken and mix until very much covered. At that point fill every wonton cup with a tablespoon or two of chicken, and after that top with a spot of blue cheddar. Return wonton cups to broiler and cook for another 5-10 minutes, or until cheddar is delicate and melty. Take out and top with cut scallions, and serve warm. These are best served right away.

NUTRITION PER SERVING:
Calories: 254 Carbs: 29g Fat: 4g Protein: 20g

Crab Salad in Crisp Wonton Cups

Total: 35min Prep: 25min Cook: 10min, Servings: 6

Ingredients

- **For the Wonton Cups:**
- Nonstick cooking spray
- 18 - wonton wrappers, thawed
- 2 - teaspoons canola oil
- ¼ - teaspoon salt
- **For the dressing:**
- 1 - teaspoon lime zest
- 2 - tablespoons fresh lime juice
- ¼ - teaspoons salt
- 1/8 - teaspoon black pepper
- ½ - teaspoon dried hot red pepper flakes
- 2 - tablespoons olive oil
- **For the salad:**
- ½ - pound lump crabmeat, picked over
- 1 - stalk celery, finely diced
- ½ - cup finely diced mango
- ¼ - cup thinly sliced scallions
- 2 - tablespoons coarsely chopped fresh cilantro leaves

Instructions:

- Preheat the stove to 375 degrees F. Splash 2 little biscuit tins with cooking shower.
- Brush the wonton wrappers with oil, and spot every wrapper into a segment of a little biscuit tin. Tenderly press every wrapper into the tin and organize with the goal that it frames a cup shape. The wrapper will cover itself and stick up out of the cup. Sprinkle with salt and prepare for 8 to 10mints, until seared and fresh. Take out from the tin and enable wrappers to cool.
- In the meantime whisk together the get-up-and-go, lime juice, salt, pepper, and pepper pieces. Include the oil and race until very much joined.
- In a medium bowl, hurl together the crabmeat, celery, mango, scallion, and cilantro. Add dressing and hurl to join. Fill each cup with the crab plate of mixed greens and serve.

NUTRITION PER SERVING:

Calories: 230 Carbs: 24g Fat: 12g Protein: 8g

Skinny Meatloaf Muffins with Barbecue Sauce

Prep Time: 15mints, Bake Time: 40mints, SERVES: 2

Ingredients:
- 1 - package (~1.25 pounds) 99% fat-free ground turkey breast
- 1 - slice whole wheat or multigrain bread
- 1 - cup onions, finely diced
- 1 - egg,
- 2 - tablespoons Worcestershire sauce
- ½ - cup Sweet barbecue sauce
- ¼ - teaspoon salt
- Fresh ground pepper, to taste
- **For Topping:**
- ⅓ - cup Sweet barbecue sauce

Instructions
- Preheat stove to 350 degrees. Coat a normal (12-cup) biscuit container with cooking shower. Since this formula makes 9 meatloaf biscuits, you'll just fill 9, not 12. Put in a safe spot.
- To make bread morsels: Toast 1 cut entire wheat or multigrain bread. Spot in blender and heartbeat until made into morsels.
- In an enormous bowl, including ground turkey, bread pieces, onions, egg, Worcestershire sauce, ½ cup grill sauce, salt, and pepper. Utilizing your hands or an enormous spoon, completely combine until very much mixed.
- Add meatloaf blend to the 9 biscuit cups, smoothing out the tops. Top every meatloaf biscuit with ¾ tablespoon grill sauce and spread equally over top.
- Heat for 40mints. Run a blade around every biscuit to slacken it from dish. Take it out to a serving plate.

NUTRITION PER SERVING:
Calories 115, Carbs 18g, Sugars 3g, Fat 2.4g, Protein 18g

Meatloaf Cupcakes with Mashed Potato Frosting

PREP TIME: 30mins COOK TIME: 20mins , Servings: 6

INGREDIENTS

MEATLOAF CUPCAKES:

- 1.3 - lb 93% lean ground turkey
- 1 - cup grated zucchini,
- 2 - tbsp onion, minced
- ½ - cup seasoned breadcrumbs
- ¼ - cup ketchup
- 1 - egg
- 1 - tsp kosher salt

SKINNY MASHED POTATO "FROSTING":

- 1 - lb about 2 medium Yukon gold potatoes, peeled and cubed
- 2 - large garlic cloves, peeled and halved
- 2 - tbsp fat free sour cream
- 2 - tbsp fat free chicken broth
- 1 - tbsp skim milk
- ½ - tbsp light butter
- kosher salt to taste
- dash of fresh ground pepper
- 2 - tbsp fresh thyme

INSTRUCTIONS

- Put the potatoes and garlic in a big pot with salt and enough water to cover and boil it. Spread and low the heat; stew for 20mints.
- Return potatoes and garlic to the container. Include acrid cream and remaining fixings.
- Utilizing a masher or blender, squash until smooth.
- Season with salt and pepper to taste.
- In the interim, preheat the broiler to 350°.
- Line a biscuit tin with foil liners.
- In a huge bowl, blend the turkey, zucchini, onion, breadcrumbs, ketchup, egg, and salt.
- Spot meatloaf blends into biscuit tins filling them to the top, ensuring they are level at the top.
- Prepare revealed for 18 to 20mints or until cooked through.
- Take out from tins and spot onto a preparing dish.
- Pipe the "icing" onto the meatloaf cupcakes and serve.

NUTRITION PER SERVING:

Calories: 240.7, Carb: 24.5g, Protein: 18.1g, Fat: 8.5g, Sugar: 4.2g

Swiss Chard Wraps With Chicken and Sweet Potato

Prep Time: 10mins Cook Time: 25mins , SERVES: 2

INGREDIENTS

- 2 - medium sweet potatoes, cut into 1-inch cubes
- 1 - teaspoon olive oil
- 1/4 teaspoon paprika
- Salt
- Pepper
- 1 - small chicken breast (about 8 oz, bone-in, skin-on)
- 4 - Swiss chard leaves, stems trimmed
- 1 - cup canned chickpeas, rinsed and drained
- ½ - medium avocado, thinly sliced
- 1 - teaspoon tahini
- Juice of 1 lime

Instructions:

- Warmth stove to 450° and line an enormous sheet container with material paper. Toss sweet potatoes with oil on a sheet dish. Season with paprika, salt, and pepper, and spread in an even layer.
- Season chicken on all sides with salt and pepper and spot on a sheet container with sweet potatoes. Broil 25 to 30mints, until chicken is cooked through and a thermometer embedded in the center peruses 165° and sweet potatoes are delicate. Cool marginally, at that point bone chicken and daintily cut meat and skin.
- Fill a huge skillet or pot with 3 crawls of water and heat to the point of boiling. Include salt.
- Fill a bowl with frosted water. Whiten Swiss chard leaves each in turn: Submerge in bubbling water 15seconds, until brilliant green. Move to ice water for 1 moment. Dry completely with paper towels.
- In another bowl, pound chickpeas, avocado, tahini, and lime juice.
- For each wrap, spread 1/4 chickpea-avocado blend down the focus of chard. Top with 1/4 chicken and sweet potato. Wrap firmly.
- Give remains a chance to cool totally before putting away in a hermetically sealed holder in the ice chest.

NUTRITION PER SERVING:

Calories 499, Fat 20g, Carbs 53g, Sugar 10g, Protein 31g.

Smashed Chickpea and Avocado Toast

Prep Time: 10mins Cook Time: 0mins , SERVES: 1

INGREDIENTS

- ½ - cup canned chickpeas, rinsed and drained
- 2 - tablespoons nutritional yeast flakes
- ½ - teaspoon olive oil
- 1 - pinch curry powder
- Salt
- Pepper
- 2 - slices 100-percent whole wheat bread, toasted
- ½ - medium ripe avocado
- ½ - lime, juiced
- 1 - tablespoon fresh parsley, chopped
- 1 - baby radish, thinly sliced

Instructions:

- In a bowl, gently pound chickpeas, yeast, oil, curry powder, and salt and pepper with a fork. The gap between toast cuts, spreading uniformly.
- In a similar little bowl, pound avocado, lime juice, and parsley. Spread over chickpea blend.
- Top with cut radishes and increasingly salt and pepper.

NUTRITION PER SERVING:

Calories 511, Fat 17g, Carbs 66g, Sugar 11g, Protein 21g.

Chickpea Fajita Bowl

Prep Time: 10mins Cook Time: 0mins , SERVES: 1

INGREDIENTS

- ¼ - cup plain 2-percent-fat Greek yogurt
- ¼ - lime, zest and juice, divided
- Salt
- Pepper
- 2 - teaspoons olive oil
- 1 - small yellow onion, sliced thin
- 1 - small bell pepper, cored and sliced thin
- 2 - cloves garlic
- ¼ - teaspoon chili powder
- 1 - cup canned chickpeas, rinsed and drained
- ¼ - medium-size ripe avocado, chopped into rough 1/2-inch pieces
- 2 - tablespoons salsa

Instructions:

- In a bowl, mix together yogurt, pizzazz (whenever wanted), and squeeze. Season with salt and pepper. Put in a safe spot.
- In a big skillet over medium warmth, heat olive oil. Include onion and ringer pepper. Season with salt and pepper. Cook, mixing until vegetables are still somewhat firm, around 5mints.
- Include garlic and bean stew powder and cook, blending, until fragrant, around 1 moment.
- Include chickpeas. Cook, mixing until warmed through, around 2mints.
- Top with lime yogurt, avocado, and salsa.

NUTRITION PER SERVING:

Calories 506, Fat 21g, Carbs 63g, Sugar 18g, Protein 21g.

Tuna, Barley, and Herb Salad With Lemon Vinaigrette

Prep Time: 10mins Cook Time: 0mins , SERVES: 1

INGREDIENTS
- 1 - lemon, zest and juice
- 1 - tablespoon Dijon mustard
- 1 - tablespoon olive oil
- 1 - teaspoon honey
- Salt
- Pepper
- 1 - can (5-oz) tuna in water, drained
- 1 - cup cooked barley
- 1 - small bell pepper, cored and chopped
- 2 - tablespoons fresh parsley, chopped
- 1 - tablespoon fresh mint, chopped
- 1 - tablespoon fresh basil, chopped

Instructions:
- In a bowl, whisk together get-up-and-go, juice, Dijon, oil, and nectar. Season with salt and pepper. Add fish and blend to cover. Include remaining fixings and hurl.
- Serve cold or at room temperature.

NUTRITION PER SERVING:
Calories 506, Fat 16g, Carbs 64g, Sugar 14g, Protein 30g.

Arugula Salad With Black Beans, Barley, Strawberry, and Feta
Prep Time: 10mins Cook Time: 0mins , SERVES: 1

INGREDIENTS
- 1 - lime, zest and juice
- 2 - teaspoons olive oil
- Salt
- Pepper
- 3 - cups baby arugula, loosely packed
- ¾ - cup canned black beans, rinsed and drained
- ½ - cup cooked hulled barley
- 2 - ounces feta, crumbled
- 6 - medium strawberries, cored and thinly sliced

Instructions:
- In a bowl, whisk together pizzazz squeeze, and oil. Season with salt and pepper. Add remaining fixings and toss to cover.
- Serve quickly, or refrigerate until serving.

NUTRITION PER SERVING:
Calories 525, Fat 23g, Carbs 64g, Sugar 8g, Protein 23g.

Cheese, Crackers, Fruit, and Egg

Prep Time: 5mins Cook Time: 0mins , SERVES: 1

INGREDIENTS
- 1 - medium apple Squeeze of lemon juice
- 10 - shredded wheat crackers
- 1 - cup cherry tomatoes, halved
- 2 - hard-boiled eggs, halved (store-bought or made ahead of time)
- ½ - ounce cheddar, sliced

Instructions:
- Center and cut apple, at that point shower with lemon juice to avert sautéing.
- Consolidate all fixings in a hermetically sealed compartment or lunchbox.
- Spread and refrigerate until prepared to serve.

NUTRITION PER SERVING:
Calories 414, Fat 18g, Carbs 47g, Sugar 24g, Protein 20g

Pita and Carrots with Hummus-Yogurt Dip

Prep Time: 10mins Cook Time: 0mins , SERVES: 4

INGREDIENTS

- 1/3 - cup plain 2-percent-fat Greek yogurt
- 3 - tablespoons hummus
- 1 - scallion, thinly sliced
- 1 - teaspoon olive oil
- Salt
- Pepper
- 1 - whole wheat pita pocket, cut in triangles
- 2 - carrots, cut in matchsticks

Instructions:

- In a little bowl, mix together yogurt, hummus, scallion, and olive oil. Season with salt and pepper.
- Spoon yogurt-hummus dunk into the edge of a sealed shut compartment or lunchbox. Fill the rest of the holder with pita triangles and carrots.
- Spread and refrigerate until prepared to serve.

NUTRITION PER SERVING:
Calories 412, Fat1 2g, Carbs 61g, Sugar 10g, Protein 20g.

Apple Salad with Chickpeas

Prep Time: 7mins Cook Time: 23mins , SERVES: 1

INGREDIENTS

- 2 - teaspoons olive oil
- 1 - teaspoon apple cider vinegar
- 1 - pinch cumin
- Salt
- Pepper
- 3 - cups kale, roughly chopped
- 1 - cup canned chickpeas, rinsed and drained
- ½ - medium apple, cored and chopped
- ½ - cup sliced cucumber

Instructions:

- In a medium bowl, blend together oil, vinegar, and cumin. Season with salt and pepper. Include kale and back rub vinaigrette into the kale until leaves begin to relax, around 2mints.
- Add remaining fixings and hurl to cover.
- Move to a sealed shut holder or lunchbox. Spread and refrigerate until prepared to serve

NUTRITION PER SERVING:*Calories 445, Fat 16g, Carbs 65g, Sugar 26g, Protein 21g.*

Chickpea, Avocado, and Egg Wrap

Prep Time: 5mins Cook Time: 20mins , SERVES: 2

INGREDIENTS

- 1 - cup kale, thinly sliced
- 1 - teaspoon olive oil
- ½ - teaspoon apple cider vinegar
- 1 - pinch cumin
- Salt
- Pepper
- ¼ - cup canned chickpeas, rinsed and drained
- 2 - tablespoons plain 2-percent-fat Greek yogurt
- 1 - whole wheat tortilla (10 inches)
- 1 - hard-boiled egg (store-bought or made ahead), thinly slice
- ¼ - avocado, thinly sliced

Instruction:

- In a medium bowl, consolidate kale, oil, vinegar, and cumin. Season with salt and pepper. Back rub vinaigrette into the kale until leaves begin to mollify, around 2mints.
- In a little bowl, utilize a fork to crush chickpeas with yogurt. Season with salt and pepper.
- To gather wrap: Spread chickpea-yogurt blend over a tortilla. Top with kale, egg, and avocado.
- Move to an impenetrable compartment or lunchbox. Spread and refrigerate until prepared to serve.

NUTRITION PER SERVING:*Calories 483, Fat 19g, Carbs 55g, Sugar 9g, Protein 23g.*

Tuna Salad with Crackers and Red Pepper Slices

Prep Time: 10mins Cook Time: 0mins , SERVES: 1

INGREDIENTS

- 1 - can (5 ounces) tuna in water, drained
- 1 - scallion, thinly sliced
- 2 - tablespoons hummus
- 1 - teaspoon olive oil
- 1 - pinch paprika
- Salt
- Pepper
- 20 - shredded wheat crackers
- 1 - small bell pepper, cored and sliced

Instructions:

- In a little bowl, blend together fish, scallion, hummus, olive oil, and paprika, separating pieces of fish. Season with salt and pepper.
- Spoon fish serving of mixed greens plunges into the edge of a sealed shut compartment or lunchbox. Fill the rest of the holder with saltines and ringer pepper cuts.
- Spread and refrigerate until prepared to serve.

NUTRITION PER SERVING:
Calories: 455, Fat 17g, Carbs 43g, Sugar 5g, Protein 34g.

Chicken, Cheddar, and Refried Bean Wrap

Prep Time: 20mins Cook Time: 0mins , SERVES: 6

INGREDIENTS

- 1 - cup loosely packed baby spinach
- 1 - pinch chili powder Squeeze of lime juice
- 1/3 - cup vegetarian refried beans
- 1 - whole wheat tortilla (10 inches)
- 3 - ounces shredded rotisserie chicken
- ¼ - avocado, sliced
- ½ - ounce cheddar, thinly sliced

Instructions:

- In a little bowl, hurl spinach with bean stew powder and lime juice.
- To gather wrap: Spread refried beans over the tortilla, at that point top with chicken, avocado, cheddar, and spinach.
- Spread and refrigerate until prepared to serve.
- Discretionary: Before serving, warm enclose by a panini press or toaster broiler.

NUTRITION PER SERVING:

Calories 487, Fat 17g, Carbs 49g, Sugar 4g, Protein 34g.

Greek Chicken Salad with Pita

Prep Time: 25mins Cook Time: 10mins , SERVES: 1

INGREDIENTS

- 3 - ounces shredded rotisserie chicken
- ½ - cup cherry tomatoes, halved
- ½ - cup chopped cucumber
- 2 - tablespoons kalamata olives, chopped
- 1 - ounce feta, crumbled
- 1 - teaspoon olive oil
- 1 - teaspoon apple cider vinegar
- 1 - pinch paprika
- Salt
- Pepper
- 1 whole wheat pita, cut in triangles

Instructions:

- In an impermeable compartment or lunchbox, toss together all fixings with the exception of pita. Settle pita triangles next to serving of mixed greens in the holder.
- Spread and refrigerate until prepared to serve.

NUTRITION PER SERVING:
Calories 433, Fat 16g, Carbs 46g, Sugar 5g, Protein 31g

Chicken Bacon Ranch Wonton Cupcakes

Prep Time: 5mins Cook Time: 10mins, SERVES: 4

INGREDIENTS:

- 1 - lb uncooked boneless, skinless chicken breasts
- 1 - tablespoon ranch seasoning
- 2 - teaspoons canola oil
- 5 - slices center cut bacon, cooked crisp and chopped
- ¾ - cup yogurt-based ranch dressing
- 24 - wonton wrappers
- 4 - oz 2% shredded sharp cheddar

Instructions:

- Preheat the stove to 375. Softly fog 12 cups in a standard biscuit/cupcake tin with cooking shower and put in a safe spot.
- Spot the uncooked chicken tenders into a Ziploc pack and sprinkle with the farm flavoring. Seal the pack and shake/rub until the chicken is covered with the flavoring.
- Bring the canola oil over medium warmth in a medium estimated skillet. At the point when the oil is hot, include the chicken pieces and blend them around to cover with oil. Orchestrate them into a solitary layer and cook for 5 to 7mints, flipping every so often, until the chicken fingers are cooked through. Take out the chicken to a cutting board and slash into little pieces.
- Spot the hacked chicken into a blending bowl and mix in the slashed bacon and farm dressing until all-around joined.
- Drive a wonton wrapper into the base of every one of the splashed cups in the biscuit tin. Utilizing the portion of the chicken blend, spoon uniformly into the wonton wrappers. Sprinkle about portion of the destroyed cheddar equitably over the highest point of each cup. Press another wonton wrapper on top and rehash the layering ventures with the staying chicken blend and destroyed cheddar.
- Prepare for 18 to 20mints until the wontons are brilliant dark colored and the substance are warmed through. Take out the biscuit tin from the stove and permit to cool for 2 to 3mints before expelling from the tin.

NUTRITION PER SERVING:
Calories 152, Carbs 10g, Sugars 1g, Fat 6g, Protein 14g.

SESAME CHICKEN WONTON CUPS

Prep Time: 45mins Cook Time: 55mins , SERVES: 4

INGREDIENTS

- 8 - Ounces boneless, skinless chicken breast
- cooking spray
- 24 - Wonton wrappers, about 6 oz.
- 2 - Tablespoons tahini
- 2 - Tablespoons soy sauce
- 2 - Tablespoons pure maple syrup, dark or amber
- 2 - Tablespoons mayonnaise
- ½ - Cup thinly sliced snow peas
- ½ - Cup shredded carrot
- ½ - Cup thinly sliced scallions
- 2 Tablespoons chopped basil
- black sesame seeds for garnish, optional

INSTRUCTIONS

- Spot chicken bosom in a medium skillet and spread with virus faucet water. Spot over high warmth and bring to a stew. Decrease warmth to keep up a delicate stew and cook until the chicken is never again pink in the inside and cooked through, 8 to 12mints, contingent upon the thickness of the meat. Evacuate the chicken and let cool. Cut chicken into little solid shapes.
- In the meantime, preheat stove to 350°F. Coat two 12cup small scale biscuit tins with cooking splash. Cut corners off wonton wrappers to make an octagonal shape. Tenderly press wrapper down into each cup. Softly spritz wrappers with cooking shower. Move the dish to the broiler and heat until the wrappers are beginning to turn brilliant dark-colored and are firm and gurgling 10 to 14mints. Let cool totally.
- Whisk tahini, soy or tamari, maple syrup and mayonnaise in a medium bowl until smooth. Blend in the chicken and refrigerate until chilly, 40mints to 60mints.
- Mix snow peas, carrot, scallions and herbs into the chicken blend. Partition the chicken serving of mixed greens among wonton cups, around 2 inadequate tablespoons each. Topping with sesame seeds, if utilizing. Serve right away.

NUTRITION PER SERVING: *CALORIES: 54, SUGAR: 1g FAT: 2g CARB: 6g PROTEIN: 3g*

Chicken Broccoli Alfredo Wonton

Prep Time: 35mins Cook Time: 35mins , SERVES: 4

INGREDIENTS:
- 1 ½ - teaspoons olive oil
- 1 - cup broccoli florets, chopped small
- 2 - cups cooked shredded
- 1 - cup light Alfredo sauce
- ½ - teaspoon Italian seasoning
- 1/8 - teaspoon black pepper
- 24 - wonton wrappers
- 1 ½ - cup shredded 2% Mozzarella cheese
- 1 - tablespoon grated Parmesan cheese

Instructions:
- Preheat the broiler to 375. Daintily fog 12 cups in a standard biscuit/cupcake tin with a cooking splash and put in a safe spot.
- Take out the oil into a skillet and bring over medium warmth. Include the broccoli and cook for 5mints or until broccoli is delicate, mixing every so often.
- Move the broccoli to a blending bowl and consolidate with the chicken, alfredo sauce, Italian flavoring, and pepper. Mix until very much consolidated.
- Drive a wonton wrapper into the base of every one of the splashed cups in the biscuit tin. Utilizing a portion of the chicken blend, spoon equitably into the wonton wrappers. Sprinkle about a large portion of the Mozzarella cheddar equitably over the highest point of each cup. Press another wonton wrapper on top and rehash the layering ventures with the staying chicken blend and Mozzarella cheddar.
- Whenever complete, sprinkle ¼ teaspoon of Parmesan cheddar over the highest point of every wonton cup.
- Heat for 18 to 20mints until brilliant darker.

NUTRITION PER SERVING:
Calories 130, Carbs 9g, Sugars 1g, Fat 5g, Protein 13g

Crunchy Taco Cups

Prep Time: 20mins Cook Time: 12mins , SERVES: 4

Ingredients
- 1 lb - lean ground beef, browned and drained

- 1 - envelope (3 tablespoons) taco seasoning
- 1 - (10-oz) can Ro-Tel Diced Tomatoes and Green Chiles, drained
- 1 ½ - cups sharp cheddar cheese, shredded
- 24 - wonton wrappers

Instructions

- Preheat stove to 375 degrees F. Liberally covers a standard size biscuit tin with nonstick cooking splash.
- Consolidate cooked meat, taco flavoring, and tomatoes in a bowl and mix to join. Line each cup of arranged biscuit tin with a wonton wrapper. Include 1.5 tablespoons taco blend. Top with 1 tablespoon of cheddar. Press down and include another layer of the wonton wrapper, taco blend, and a last layer of cheddar.
- Prepare at 375 for 11-13 minutes until cups are warmed through and edges are brilliant.

NUTRITION PER SERVING:

Calories 463, Carbs 32g, Sugars 2g, Fat 18g, Protein 39g

Gastric Sleeve Dinner Recipes

ROASTED KIELBASA AND CABBAGE

PREP TIME: 15mins COOK TIME: 35mins , SERVINGS: 4

INGREDIENTS

- **MUSTARD VINAIGRETTE**
- ¼ - cup olive oil
- 2 - Tbsp red wine vinegar
- 1 - Tbsp stone ground or whole grain mustard
- 1 - small clove garlic, crushed or minced
- ¼ - tsp salt
- Freshly cracked pepper
- **ROASTED KIELBASA AND VEGETABLES**
- ½ - lb kielbasa
- 1 - lb baby red potatoes
- ½ - head cabbage
- 2 - Tbsp olive oil, divided
- Pinch of salt and pepper
- Handful chopped fresh parsley

INSTRUCTIONS

- Preheat the broiler to 400ºF. In a bit bowl whisk collectively the olive oil, red wine vinegar, mustard, squashed garlic, salt, and crisply cut up pepper for the vinaigrette. Put the French dressing in a secure spot.
- Cut the kielbasa into 1/4 inch thick. Wash the potatoes properly and cut them into 1/4 inch adjusts also. Set the kielbasa and potatoes on a big heating sheet and sprinkle with 1 Tbsp olive oil. Toss the kielbasa and potatoes in the oil till they're all around included and the outside of the heating sheet is likewise canvassed in oil. Sprinkle a touch of salt and pepper over top.
- Take any dirty or harmed leaves out from the cabbage. Cut the stem off the cabbage, at that factor reduce it down the center. Hold one half for an alternate formulation. Cut the staying half into 1-inch extensive cuts. Cut every cut into portions. Spot the cabbage portions on the heating sheet with the kielbasa and potatoes, settling them down so they are laying level at the getting ready sheet.

- Brush the staying 1 Tbsp olive oil over the outdoor of the cabbage pieces and consist of the closing squeeze of salt and pepper to each.
- Cook the kielbasa, potatoes, and cabbage within the preheated broiler for 20mins. Take the heating sheet out from the range and carefully turn the kielbasa, potatoes, and cabbage pieces. The cabbage may additionally self-destruct a chunk as it's flipped, that's o.K.. Return the heating sheet to the broiler and dish for an extra 10-15mints, or until the cabbage is sensitive and the rims are particularly darkish-colored and fresh. The kielbasa and potato cuts need to be all-around seared.
- Take the preparing sheet out from the broiler and top with new slashed parsley and a sprinkle of the mustard vinaigrette. Serve heat.

NUTRITION PER SERVING:
Calories: 269 Carbs: 19g Fat: 13g Protein: 22g

SHEET PAN SWEET AND SOUR CHICKEN

PREP TIME: 20mins COOK TIME: 40mins , SERVINGS: 6

INGREDIENTS

- 1 - large onion
- 2 - green bell peppers
- 1 - red bell pepper
- 20 - oz can pineapple chunks
- 2 - boneless skinless chicken breasts (about 1.25 lb.)
- 2 - Tbsp cooking oil
- ¼ - tsp garlic powder
- ½ - tsp ground ginger
- Salt and Pepper to taste
- ¼ - cup ketchup
- ¼ - cup brown sugar
- 1/3 - cup rice or apple cider vinegar
- 1.5 - Tbsp soy sauce
- 1.5 - Tbsp cornstarch
- 3 - green onions, sliced
- 6 - cups cooked rice

INSTRUCTIONS

- Preheat the broiler to 400ºF. Cut the onion, ringer peppers, and chicken bosoms into one-inch pieces. Channel the pineapple well, holding the juice for the sauce. Spot the onion, chime pepper, chicken, and pineapple lumps on an enormous sheet container in a solitary layer. Utilize two sheets, if necessary, to keep the chicken and vegetables from heaping over one another. They need a little space to darker effectively.
- Sprinkle the cooking oil over the fixings on the sheet skillet, trailed by the garlic powder, ground ginger, and a squeeze or two of salt and pepper. Hurl the chicken, chime peppers, onions, and pineapple until they are equitably covered in oil and flavors.
- Heat the chicken and vegetables in the broiler for about 40mints, or until they are somewhat cooked on the edges. Blend part of the way through the preparing time to redistribute the warmth and enable abundance dampness to dissipate.

- While the chicken and vegetables are heating, set up the sauce. In a little saucepot whisk together the held pineapple juice (around 1 cup), ketchup, dark colored sugar, vinegar, soy sauce, and cornstarch until the cornstarch is completely broken down. Warmth the blend over medium fire, mixing regularly, until it starts to stew. When it starts to stew the cornstarch will start to gel and thicken the sauce. When the sauce has thickened to a coating, expel it from the warmth and put it aside until prepared to utilize.
- At the point when the chicken and vegetables have got done with heating, take them out from the stove and pour the readied sauce over top. Blend until everything is covered in sauce.
- Serve the sweet and harsh chicken over cooked rice with cut green onions sprinkled over top.

NUTRITION PER SERVING:
Calories: 290 Carbs: 54g Fat: 5g Protein: 8g

One Sheet Pan Chicken Fried Rice

PREP TIME 5MINTS COOK TIME 15MINTS, SERVINGS: 4

Ingredients

- 2 - boneless skinless chicken breasts.
- salt and pepper, to taste
- 1 15 - ounce can peas and carrots, drained
- ½ - white onion, diced
- 2 - eggs, whisked
- 2 - cups steamed white rice
- 3 - tablespoons sesame oil
- 1/3 - cup soy sauce
- finely chopped green onions

Instructions

- Oil an enormous preparing sheet and preheat stove to 375 degrees. Mastermind chicken pieces on the dish in a solitary layer so they aren't covering and season with salt and pepper to taste. Heat for 5mints.
- Take the dish out from the stove, pour whisked eggs around the chicken pieces straightforwardly onto the container. Come back to broiler for 3-5mints until the egg is completely cooked. Utilize a fork or spatula to "scramble" the egg with the goal that it separates into little pieces.
- Include rice and peas, carrots and white onions to the container and hurl all fixings so they are equitably appropriated. Shower sesame oil and soy sauce over everything and hurl once more. Sprinkle cleaved onions over the top.
- Prepare for 5mints longer. Chicken ought to be cooked through and rice should start to darker on the base of the dish.
- Toss all fixings once again and serve right away.

NUTRITION PER SERVING:
Calories: 246 Carbs: 24g Fat: 6g Protein: 28g

Healthy Sheet Pan Chicken Fajitas

PREP TIME 10MINTS COOK TIME 20MINTS, SERVINGS: 6

Ingredients

- 3 - boneless skinless chicken breasts pounded
- 4 - bell peppers, sliced any color
- 1 - large onion, sliced
- 4 - tablespoons olive oil divided
- salt and pepper to taste
- 1 - teaspoon garlic powder
- 1 - teaspoon chili powder
- 1 - teaspoon cumin
- ½ - teaspoon cayenne pepper
- juice of 1 lime
- 8 6 - inch flour tortillas
- **Toppings:**
- light sour cream
- Salsa
- Mashed
- Chopped cilantro
- Lime wedges for squeezing

Instructions

- Preheat stove to 375 degrees and daintily oil a huge sheet skillet. Mix together garlic powder, stew powder, cumin, and cayenne pepper.
- Organize chicken bosoms on the container, shower with 2 tablespoons olive oil and rub in with your fingers on the two sides. Season liberally with salt on the two sides, at that point season chicken with blended flavors on the two sides.
- Organize cut peppers and onions on the container around the chicken bosoms. Shower with staying 2 tablespoons olive oil. Season liberally with salt.
- Prepare for 15 to 20mints until chicken is cooked through. Move chicken to a cutting board, return peppers and onions to the stove and change to BROIL for 3 to 5mints until the edges of the veggies begin to singe marginally, at that point expel from broiler.
- While veggies are searing, shower new lime squeeze over chicken at that point daintily cut into strips.

- Gather fajitas with chicken, peppers, onions, and wanted garnishes and serve right away.

NUTRITION PER SERVING:
Calories: 241 Carbs: 7g Fat: 16g Protein: 17g

SHEET PAN GARLIC TOFU & BRUSSELS SPROUT DINNER
Prep time: 15MINTS Cook Time: 30MINTS , SERVING SIZE: 4

INGREDIENTS

- 14 - ounce package of Extra Firm Organic Tofu, pressed
- 1 - pound Brussels Sprouts, cleaned and diced, approximately 2 cups prepared
- 1 - tablespoon olive oil
- 2 - tablespoon balsamic vinegar
- 1 - tablespoon minced garlic
- ¼ - teaspoon sea salt
- ¼ - teaspoon black pepper
- ½ - cup dried cranberries
- ¼ - cup pumpkin seeds
- 1 - tablespoon balsamic glaze

INSTRUCTIONS

- Preheat the broiler to 400 degrees F
- Channel the overabundance water from the holder of tofu.
- Shakers the tofu into 1-inch reduced down pieces, and press between two clean towels for 15mints to wick away extra dampness.
- Reap, clean and bones your Brussels grows.
- In a big bowl, combine the Brussels grows, oil, vinegar, and garlic. Include the salt, pepper, and tofu and Big tenderly until the tofu is all around covered.
- Splash a foil-fixed heating sheet with cooking shower.
- Put into the stove and heat for 20mints.
- After 20mints, expel from the stove and blend.
- Equally spread the pumpkin seeds and cranberries and come back to the broiler for an extra 10 minutes.
- Take out from the stove and sprinkle with balsamic coating.

NUTRITION PER SERVING:
CALORIES: 250 FAT: 2g CARB: 18g SUGAR: 13g PROTEIN: 13g

SHEET PAN CAULIFLOWER NACHOS

Prep time: 15MINTS Cook time: 20 MINTS , SERVINGS: 6

INGREDIENTS:

- 1 - head cauliflower, cut into florets
- 2 - T-spoon olive oil
- ¼ - T-spoon chili powder
- 3 - cloves garlic, minced
- ½ - T-spoon cumin
- ¼ - teaspoon smoked paprika
- Kosher salt and freshly ground black pepper,
- 6 - ounces tortilla chips
- 1 - (15-ounce) can black beans, drained and rinsed
- 1 - cup shredded cheddar cheese
- 1 - Roma tomato, diced
- 1/3 - cup guacamole, homemade
- ¼ - cup diced red onion
- 1 - jalapeno, thinly sliced
- 2 - T-spoon chopped fresh cilantro leaves

Instructions:
- Preheat stove to 425 degrees F. Softly oil a heating sheet.
- Spot cauliflower florets in a solitary layer onto the readied heating sheet. Include olive oil, garlic, cumin, bean stew powder, and paprika; season with salt and pepper, to taste. Tenderly hurl to consolidate. Spot into the stove and prepare for 12 to 14mints, or until delicate and brilliant darker.
- Blend in tortilla contributes a solitary layer. Top with dark beans and cheddar.
- Spot into the stove and prepare until warmed through and the cheddar liquefies around 5 to 6mints.
- Serve promptly; beat with tomato, guacamole, onion, jalapeno, and cilantro.

NUTRITION PER SERVING:
Calories: 404 Carbs: 5g Fat: 23g Protein: 42g

Sheet pan spicy tofu and green beans

Prep Time: 15mints Cook Time: 30mints , Servings: 4

INGREDIENTS

Spicy Marinade:

- 1 - teaspoon minced garlic
- ¼ - cup sliced scallions
- 2 - teaspoons sesame seeds, plus more for garnish
- 3 - tablespoons soy sauce
- 1 - tablespoon sesame oil
- 1 - teaspoon red pepper flakes
- ½ - teaspoon maple syrup

- 2 - tablespoons of rice wine vinegar
- 16 - ounces firm tofu, drained and pressed
- 1 - pound green beans, trimmed
- 2 - teaspoons olive oil, for oiling the pan
- Salt/pepper

INSTRUCTIONS

- Preheat the broiler to 400 degrees F.
- Flush and channel your tofu, at that point press utilizing a tofu press or envelop by paper towels and spot overwhelming books or dish on top. Let channel for in any event 10 to 15mints, this will enable the marinade to be assimilated.
- Whisk together the elements for the zesty sauce.
- Cut the tofu into triangles and spot in a solitary layer on an oiled preparing sheet. Shower with the hot sauce at that point prepares for 12mints.
- Flip tofu and sprinkle with more sauce. Add the green beans to the opposite side of the container in a solitary layer, as would be prudent. Shower with residual sauce and sprinkle with salt and pepper.
- Return back to the stove and heat until tofu is caramelized and somewhat fresh, around 12-15 minutes.
- Sprinkle with residual sesame seeds, whenever wanted, and serve.

NUTRITION PER SERVING:*Calories: 218 Carbs: 20g Fat: 11g Protein: 12g*

SHEET PAN ZUCCHINI PARMESAN

Prep Time: 15MINTS Cook Time: 25MINTS, SERVINGS: 6

INGREDIENTS:

- 1 - cup Panko
- 1/3 - cup freshly grated Parmesan cheese
- Kosher salt and freshly ground black pepper, to taste
- 2 - zucchinis, thinly sliced to 1/4-inch thick rounds
- 1/3 - cup all-purpose flour
- 2 - large eggs, beaten
- ½ - cup marinara sauce
- ½ - cup mozzarella pearls, drained
- 2 - tablespoons chopped fresh parsley leaves

Instructions:

- Preheat broiler to 400 degrees F. Daintily oil a preparing sheet or coat with nonstick shower.
- In an enormous bowl, consolidate Panko and Parmesan; season with salt and pepper, to taste. Put in a safe spot.
- Working in clumps, dig zucchini adjusts in flour, dunk into eggs, at that point dig in Panko blend, squeezing to cover.
- Spot zucchini in a solitary layer onto the readied heating sheet. Spot into stove and heat until delicate and brilliant dark-colored, around 18 to 20mints.
- Top with marinara and mozzarella.
- At that point cook for 2 to 3mints, or until the cheddar has dissolved.
- Serve quickly, embellished with parsley, whenever wanted.

NUTRITION PER SERVING:
Calories: 217 Carbs: 21g Fat: 12g Protein: 8g

Honey Garlic Chicken Sheet Pan Dinner

Prep Time 15mints Cook Time 35 to 40mints, Servings: 4

Ingredients
- ¼ - cup chicken broth or water
- 1/3 - cup honey
- 6 - cloves garlic, minced
- 2 - Tbsp rice wine vinegar
- 1 - Tbsp soy sauce
- 2 - tsp garlic powder
- Salt and pepper, to taste
- 2 - large potatoes, washed and chopped into 1" pieces
- 5 to 6 - chicken legs
- 1 - broccoli crown, chopped

Instructions:
- Preheat broiler to 425 F. what's more, oil a sheet dish.
- Join the chicken soup, nectar, minced garlic, rice wine vinegar, soy sauce, and garlic powder in a blending bowl. Add hacked potatoes to the bowl and blend to cover well. Spoon potatoes onto the readied heating sheet utilizing an opened spoon so as to hold fluid in the blending bowl.
- Add chicken legs to the rest of the sauce in the bowl and coat well. Spot the covered chicken over the potatoes and pour remaining sauce over chicken legs in the skillet. Season chicken legs with salt and pepper.
- Add hacked broccoli to the sheet skillet.
- Prepare for 35 to 40mints or until chicken is never again pink and squeezes run clear.
- Serve Honey Garlic Chicken Sheet Pan Dinner, as a simple one-dish supper!

NUTRITION PER SERVING:
Calories: 237 Carbs: 5g Fat: 11g Protein: 27g

One Pan Parmesan-Crusted Chicken with Broccoli

PREP TIME: 5mins COOK TIME: 30mins , Servings: 6

INGREDIENTS
- 2 - tablespoons olive oil

- 6 to 7- ounce boneless, skinless chicken breasts
- 12 - ounces fresh or frozen broccoli florets
- 1 - teaspoon Kosher Salt
- ¼ - tsp garlic powder
- 2 - garlic cloves, minced
- ½ - cup freshly grated Parmesan cheese
- ¼ - cup chopped fresh parsley

INSTRUCTIONS

- Preheat the broiler to 425°F. Oil a rimmed preparing sheet with 1 tablespoon of the olive oil.
- Organize the chicken bosoms in the focal point of the readied preparing sheet. Orchestrate the broccoli around the chicken.
- Shower the broccoli with the staying 1 tablespoon olive oil and sprinkle everything with salt and garlic powder.
- Prepare until the chicken bosoms are cooked through and a thermometer embedded in the thickest part enlists 160°F, 25 to 30mints.
- In a little bowl, consolidate the garlic, Parmesan, and parsley.
- Top every chicken bosom with a portion of the blends. Sear until the cheddar is softened and the broccoli is profoundly cooked 3mints.
- Take the container out from the broiler, tent with foil, and let rest for 5mints. Serve warm.

NUTRITION PER SERVING:
Calories: 334 Carbs: 4g Fat: 13g Protein: 51g

Beef Roast with Winter Vegetables

Prep Time 10mints Cook Time 3hrs, Servings: 6

Ingredients

- 2 - lb. chuck or round roast
- 2 - cups baby carrots or carrot sticks
- 2 - large parsnips, peeled and cut into chunks
- 4 - medium sweet potatoes
- 1 - acorn squash, peeled, seeded and cubed
- 1 - teaspoon Italian seasoning
- Drizzles of olive oil and balsamic vinegar
- Salt and pepper, to taste

Instructions:

- Preheat the broiler to 400 F.
- Spot the hamburger cook in the focal point of a medium-sized broiling container. Toss the carrots, parsnips, sweet potatoes, and squash around the hamburger cook. Season with Italian flavoring at that point showers olive oil and balsamic vinegar over the top.
- Spread the cooking container and spot in the preheated broiler. Cook for around two hours, contingent upon the size of the meal.
- Addition a meat thermometer and cook until 140 F for medium to 165 F for all-around done.
- In the event that you favor a juicier, however, less crusted dish, cook it at 325 F for around three hours, or until the meat thermometer peruses 145 F, for medium-well.
- Serve hamburger cook with winter vegetables as may be, or with a straightforward side plate of mixed greens.

NUTRITION PER SERVING:
Calories: 295 Carbs: 28g Fat: 17g Protein: 3g

Sheet Pan Chicken Stirfry

Prep Time: 5mints Cook Time: 30mints, Servings: 6

Ingredients

- Stir fry sauce
- 2 - Tbs brown sugar
- 2 - Tbs oyster sauce
- 2 - Tbs soy sauce
- 1 - Tbs Hoisin
- 1 ½ - lb chicken breast cut into thin strips
- 5 - cups stir fry veggies

Instructions

- Preheat broiler to 350 degrees
- In a medium-sized bowl, combine pan fried food sauce and whisk all fixings together.
- Coat chicken in sauce, and
- Dump chicken on a sheet skillet, and include the veggies in.

- Blend them together to cover the veggies, and ensure it is one, even, layer on the sheet dish.
- Heat for 30mints until chicken is cooked through

NUTRITION PER SERVING:
Calories: 248kcal Carb: 25g Protein: 29g Fat: 3g Sugar: 3g

HONEY & SOY GLAZED RADISHES

PREP TIME: 10MINS COOK TIME: 15MINS , SERVES: 2

Ingredients:
- 1 - bunch of radishes, with greens
- 1 ½ - tablespoons olive oil
- ¼ - cup honey
- 2 - tablespoons soy sauce
- 1 - tablespoon unseasoned rice vinegar
- 1 - cup cooked white rice
- Fried eggs for serving

Instructions:
- Separate the greens from the radishes and generally slash them. Cut huge radishes into equal parts and keep littler radishes entirely.
- Warm the oil in an enormous skillet over medium-high heat. Include the radishes and cook, blending frequently until daintily sautéed and fresh delicate, about 10mints. Include the nectar and lessen the warmth to medium. Cook, mixing regularly until the radishes are coated, around 3 to 5mints. Include the soy sauce and cook until syrupy, about 5mints longer. Blend in the rice vinegar and radish greens, increment the warmth to high and keep on cooking until the greens are shriveled and the vast majority of the fluid has vanished.
- Present with cooked white rice and singed eggs.

NUTRITION PER SERVING: *Calories: 229 Carbs: 2g Fat: 13g Protein: 24g*

Skillet Salmon With Tomato Quinoa

Prep Time: 20mins Cook Time: 15mints , Servings: 1

INGREDIENTS

- 2 - teaspoons canola oil
- 3 - cloves garlic, finely chopped
- 1 - cup cooked quinoa
- ¾ - cup canned diced tomatoes
- ¼ - teaspoon paprika
- Salt
- Pepper
- 1 - cup loosely packed baby spinach
- 2 - tablespoons fresh basil, chopped
- 1 - salmon filet

Instructions:

- Warm stove to 425°.
- In a little ovenproof skillet over medium warmth, heat oil. Include garlic and cook, mixing, until fragrant, around 1 moment. Include quinoa, tomatoes, and paprika. Season with salt and pepper. Cook, mixing until warmed through. Include spinach and basil and blend to wither.
- Season salmon generously with salt and pepper. Spot salmon over the quinoa blend. Move to broiler and meal 8 to 12mints for medium-uncommon, 12 to 18mints for all-around done.
- Give scraps a chance to cool totally before putting away in a water/air proof compartment in the refrigerator.

NUTRITION PER SERVING:
Calories: 503, Fat 18g, Carbs 54g, Sugar 6g, Protein 30g.

Salmon Soba Noodle Miso BowlPrint

Prep Time: 5mins Cook Time: 15mints , Servings: 1

Ingredients
- Salt
- 1 - ounce dried soba noodles
- 1 - tablespoon white miso paste
- 3 - cups of filtered water
- 2 - teaspoons mirin, optional
- 4 to 5 - cauliflower florets
- 3 - ounce filet of wild-caught salmon
- ½ - baby bok choy, ends trimmed
- Sesame seeds

Instructions:
- Bring a medium pot of salted water, set over medium warmth, to a moderate bubble. Include the soba noodles and cook for around 4 to 5mints (the bundle consistently says like 10 minutes and that is WAY excessively long, so give it a taste at the 4mints imprint to ensure it's everything great). Expel when it's exceptionally still somewhat firm since we'll be cooking it again toward the end. Channel and put in a safe spot.
- In a similar void medium pot (no compelling reason to wash it out, excessively apathetic!) you cooked the soba noodles, include the miso glue and water. Turn the warmth to medium and give it a blend until the miso glue has broken down around 5 minutes. Include around 1/2 teaspoon of salt and mirin. Blend and give it a taste; modify the salt as indicated by taste. Turn the warmth to low and save.
- Preheat the broiler to 300 degrees F. Sprinkle the salmon on the two sides with a couple of portions of salt. Warmth the olive oil in a little sauté container set over medium-high heat. At the point when the oil is flickering, include the cauliflower florets and cook for 2 to 3mints. Expel and put in a safe spot. Include a teaspoon or two a greater amount of oil to the skillet. At the point when the oil was hot, include the salmon skin-side down; cook for 2 to 3mints. Flip the salmon to the opposite side and move to the broiler to cook for an extra 5mints.
- In the interim, including the bok choy, saved soba noodles, and cauliflower to the miso blend, cook for an extra 2mints until the bok choy turns somewhat delicate and the shading goes splendid green. Spoon into a bowl and top with the salmon.

NUTRITION PER SERVING:
Calories: 450 Carbs: 36g Fat: 20g Protein: 32g

Apple Cider Glazed Chicken Breast with Carrots

TOTAL TIME 6hrs 45mints, SERVING SIZE: 2

Ingredients:

- 2 - boneless skin-on chicken breasts
- 2 - cups apple cider
- 4 - Whole peppercorns
- 2 - small bunches of fresh sage
- ½ - teaspoon salt
- 2 - tablespoons olive oil
- salt and pepper, to taste
- 4 - carrots, peeled and sliced
- 1 - tablespoon butter

Instructions

- To start with, in all probability, your boneless skin-on chicken bosom still has the tenderloin connected. Expel (it's the additional piece that resembles a chicken strip). This helps the chicken cooks quicker. I solidify the tenderloins for soup or make chicken strips with them.
- In an enormous dish or bowl, include the chicken, apple juice, peppercorns, sage (torn and hacked first), and ½ teaspoon of salt. Let marinate shrouded in the cooler for at least 4hrs.
- Following 4hrs, expel the chicken and pat the chicken dry. Warm the oil in a huge skillet. At the point when the oil is hot, sprinkle the chicken with additional salt and pepper and spot it skin-side down in the container. Cook on both side until brilliant darker.
- In the mean time, strip and bones the carrots. Spot them in a microwave-safe bowl, spread with saran wrap and microwave for 1 moment.
- Take the flavors out from the apple juice, and after that pour it over the chicken once the two sides are brilliant dark-colored. Change the warmth so the apple juice goes to a stew and cook until the chicken registers 165-degrees F on a thermometer. Evacuate the chicken and put aside when done.
- When the chicken is done, turn the warmth to high and lessen the apple juice to a thick coat. Include the carrots and saute for 3 to 4mints, until fresh delicate. Include the spread before expelling them from the dish. Mix to cover the carrots

in the coating and margarine. Utilize any additional coating from the dish to brush on the chicken and serve the chicken with the carrots.

NUTRITION PER SERVING:
CALORIES: 328 FAT: 20g CARB: 39g SUGAR: 27g PROTEIN: 2g.

Stir-Fried Chicken With Corn and Millet

Prep Time: 5mins Cook Time: 15mints , Servings: 1

INGREDIENTS
- 3 - ounces boneless, skinless chicken thighs, cut into 1-inch pieces
- Salt
- Pepper
- ½ - tablespoon olive oil
- 2 - cloves garlic, sliced thin
- ½ - cup fresh corn kernels
- 2/3 - cup cooked millet
- 2 - tablespoons fresh parsley, chopped
- ¼ - lime, juiced
- ¼ - medium-size ripe avocado, chopped into ½ - inch pieces

Instructions:
- Season hen on all facets with salt and pepper. In a massive skillet over medium warmth, heat olive oil. Include chook and garlic and prepare dinner, blending sometimes, until fowl is cooked via, around 4mints.
- Include corn and prepare dinner, blending, just until it begins to mellow, round 2mints greater.
- Include millet, parsley, and juice. Cook, blending till warmed thru. Top with avocado.

NUTRITION PER SERVING:*Calories 537, Fat 20g, Carbs 66g, Sugar 5g, Protein 27g*

Chicken Chili Recipe For One

Prep Time: 10mints Cook Time: 35mints, Serves: 1

Ingredients

- 1 - tablespoon olive oil
- 1 - cup chopped onion (1/2 small onion)
- 1 - garlic clove, minced
- 1 - small red pepper, cored, seeded, and large diced
- ¼ - teaspoon chili powder
- ¼ - teaspoon ground cumin
- ½ - teaspoon kosher salt
- 1 15 - ounce can of diced tomatoes
- ½ - teaspoon dried basil
- 1 - chicken breast, cooked and chopped
- shredded cheddar cheese, optional for topping
- sour cream, optional for topping

Instructions

- Cook the onions inside the olive oil over medium-low warmness for 8 to 10mints, till the onions are translucent.
- Add the garlic and cook for 1 minute more.
- Add the pink peppers, chili powder, cumin, and salt. Cook for 1mint
- Pour the canned diced tomatoes and dried basil into the pan. Bring to a boil, and then lessen warmth to low and simmer, exposed for 15mints.
- Add the cooked, chopped hen to the pan and simmer, exposed another 5mints.
- Transfer chicken chili to a bowl and top with shredded cheddar cheese and sour cream.

NUTRITION PER SERVING:
Calories: 477kcal Carb: 21g Protein: 50g Fat: 20g Sugar: 9g.

Grilled Fig and Peach Arugula Salad with Ricotta Salata and a Black Pepper VinagrettePrint

Prep Time: 15mins Cook Time: 20mints , Servings: 2

Ingredients

Dressing:

- 3 - tablespoons good-quality olive oil
- 1 - teaspoon good balsamic vinegar
- ½ lemon from juice
- Salt
- 6 to 7 - turns freshly ground pepper

Salad:

- 4 - figs, halved
- 1 - teaspoon dark brown sugar
- Salt
- Olive oil
- Few handfuls of arugula, 2 ounces, cleaned and dried
- 1 - yellow peach, sliced
- 3 to 4 - pistachios, chopped
- 2 - slices prosciutto
- Ricotta Salata

Instructions:

- In a little bowl, including the olive oil, balsamic vinegar, lemon juice, squeeze of salt and naturally ground pepper; blend until altogether joined. Do a trial and include more salt, in the event that you like. Put in a safe spot.
- Sprinkle the figs with the dim dark colored sugar and a touch of salt. Warmth a barbecue or flame broil skillet. Whenever hot, brush with olive oil. Spot the figs on the hot flame broil, face down and cook for 1-2 minutes, until barbecue imprints show up. Expel and put in a safe spot.
- To a huge blending bowl, include the arugula. Sprinkle the leaves with salt. Include half of the dressing and delicately prepare the serving of mixed greens. Move the lettuce to your serving plate. Add the peaches to the blending bowl and hurl with a touch of dressing. Move the peaches and figs to the serving plate, masterminding anyway you like. Top with a sprinkling of pistachios, a couple of torn bits of prosciutto and slight cuts of Ricotta Salata.

NUTRITION PER SERVING:

Calories: 340 Carbs: 26g Fat: 24g Protein: 10g

Shrimp Scampi For One

PREP TIME 15mins TOTAL TIME 25mins, Serves: 1

INGREDIENTS

- ¼ - pound 21 count shrimp, about 6
- 1 - large shallot, minced
- 2 to 3 - cloves garlic, minced
- 2 - Tablespoons butter
- 3 - Tablespoons cream
- Splash of white wine (optional)
- 1/8 - teaspoon crushed red pepper flakes (optional)
- Parmesan cheese (optional)
- Salt and pepper
- Spaghetti
- ¼ - cup reserved pasta water

Instructions:

- Cook pasta as indicated by the bundle. Hold a portion of the cooking water for the sauce later. Channel the pasta and put it in a safe spot.
- Mince garlic and shallots and clean the shrimp in the event that they aren't as of now cleaned.
- Add spread to pot over medium warmth. When hot and liquefied, include the cleaned shrimp and cook for 90 seconds for every side. At that point include shallots and garlic and cook for an additional 30 seconds until delicate.
- Include a sprinkle of white wine and the squashed red pepper. Do whatever it takes not to overcook them.
- Add cream to the shrimp and blend. The sauce ought to decrease pleasantly.
- Include pasta over into the pot and blend to join. Season with salt and pepper. On the off chance that the sauce is excessively thick, include a touch of saved pasta water to thin it out. Try not to make it excessively slim, however!

NUTRITION PER SERVING:
Calories: 835 Fat 43.5g Carb 62.2g Sugars 2.4g Protein 45.5g

SAVORY OATMEAL WITH CHEDDAR AND FRIED EGG

Prep Time: 2mints Cook Time: 8mints , Serves: 1

INGREDIENTS
- ¼- cup dry quick-cooking steel-cut oats
- ¾ - cup water
- salt and pepper
- 2 - tablespoons shredded white cheddar cheese
- 1 - tsp coconut oil, divided
- ¼ - cup diced red pepper
- 2 - tablespoons finely chopped onions
- 1 - large egg
- Optional Toppings
- chopped walnuts
- sliced green onions
- Spice blend

INSTRUCTIONS
- Bring water to bubble. Include oats, diminish the warmth a little and let it cook for about 3mints until all fluid is assimilated. Mood killer warmth and mix in cheddar, a little squeeze of salt, and pepper.
- Warm a nonstick dish with ½ teaspoon of coconut oil over medium-high heat. Include vegetables and cook for 2 to 3mints, until they mollify. Spoon vegetables over cooked oats. Diminish warmth to medium.
- Include staying ½ teaspoon of oil and fry an egg. Cook until the whites are never again translucent and serve over oats.
- Top with slashed pecans, green onions, and za'atar, on the off chance that you like.

NUTRITION PER SERVING:
Calories: 307 Carbs: 31g Fat: 15g Protein: 14g

Skillet Chicken Thighs with Potato, Apple, and Spinach

Prep Time: 5mins Cook Time: 20mints , Servings: 1

INGREDIENTS
- 1 - small chicken thigh

- Salt
- Pepper
- 1 - teaspoon canola oil
- 1 - medium russet potato, cut into ½ inch cubes
- 1 - small Fuji apple, cored and cut into 6 wedges
- 1 - teaspoon fresh sage, chopped
- 1 - cup packed baby spinach

Instructions:
- Warm broiler to 400°.
- Season bird generously with salt and pepper.
- In an extensive, broiler-secure skillet over medium warmth, warmness oil. Include bird, skin side down, and prepare dinner till pores and skin crisps marginally and a few fats are rendered round 3 mints. Include potato, apple, and sage. Toss to cowl and arrange potato and apple around the skillet, making sure hen is skin side down.
- Move skillet to broiler and dish 15mints. Flip chicken, at that factor, broil 10mints extra, till potatoes and apples are delicate and chicken is cooked thru with no red within the middle.
- Return skillet to stovetop over medium-low heat. take off the chicken, consist of spinach and hurl with potatoes and apples to shrivel.
- Top vegetable mixture with chook to serve.

NUTRITION PER SERVING:
Calories 514, Fat 22g, Carbs 59g, Sugar 23g, Protein 21g.

10-MINUTE SPICY PUMPKIN CURRY CHOWDER IN A MUG

Prep Time: 4mints Cook Time: 6mints, SERVES: 1

INGREDIENTS

- 3 - tablespoons diced potatoes
- 3 - tablespoons chopped kale
- 2 - baby carrots, thinly sliced
- 2 - tablespoons corn
- ½ - cup (120ml) vegetable broth
- ¼ - cup (60g) pumpkin puree
- 1/3 - cup (80ml) unsweetened soy milk
- 2 - teaspoons maple syrup
- 1 - teaspoon curry powder
- ½ - teaspoon kosher salt
- 1/8 - teaspoon granulated garlic
- pinch of cayenne powder
- cashew cream for topping (optional)
- chopped chives for topping (optional)

INSTRUCTIONS

- Set potatoes, kale carrots, and corn into a microwave-safe mug. Pour the vegetable soup inside. Spread the mug with microwave-secure saran wrap and jab a couple of gaps on it with a blade.
- Spot mug on a plate. With your microwave at medium-high powder, microwave the vegetables for 1 to 30seconds. The energy yield of my microwave is adjusted from 1 to 10, and I set it to 7 for this development. Remove the mug from the microwave and blend the greens a bit. Microwave for a further 45seconds.
- Take the mug out, allow it to cool and pour the pumpkin, soy milk, curry, salt, garlic, and cayenne in to blend. On the alternative hand, you could combo the rest of the fixings in a one of a kind bowl and after that vacant it into the mug. Spread the mug with grasp wrap yet again.
- With the microwave at a decrease energy putting (5/10 in my microwave), cook the soup for 1 second. Take soup out and supply everything a mix with the intention that the greens cook uniformly. Rehash this level 2 extra activities.
- Give the soup a danger to rest for 2mints before consuming. This allows the veggies to finish the manner of cooking. Top with cashew cream and chives inside the event which you like.

NUTRITION PER SERVING:

Calories: 210 Carbs: 34g Fat: 6g Protein: 7g

Healthy Pita Pizza with Goat Cheese

Prep Time: 10mints Cook Time: 10mits , SERVES: 1

INGREDIENTS

- 4 - whole-wheat pitas
- 1 - small red onion
- Handful thyme sprigs
- 1 - pound tomatoes
- 2 - cups shredded mozzarella cheese
- 4 - ounces goat cheese
- Kosher salt
- Fresh ground pepper
- Olive oil (optional)

INSTRUCTIONS

- Spot a pizza stone in the broiler and preheat to 450°F.
- Spot pita straightforwardly on the stove grind and pre-heat 3 minutes for each side, at that point flip and prepare an additional 3 minutes.
- In the interim, daintily cut the red onion. Generally hack the thyme. Utilizing a serrated blade, meagerly cut the tomatoes.
- At the point when the pitas are fresh, expel them from the stove. The top each with 1/2 cup mozzarella, at that point tomatoes, onions, and thyme leaves. Include dabs of goat cheddar.
- Sprinkle generously with fit salt, particularly the tomatoes. Whenever wanted, shower with olive oil. Heat until the cheddar is softened, around 5mints. Take out from the broiler, cut into wedges, and serve.

NUTRITION PER SERVING:
Calories: 283 Carbs: 40g Fat: 9g Protein: 12g

Gastric Sleeve Soup Recipes

Beef, Mushroom and Barley Soup

Prep Time: 25mins Cook Time: 1hr 15mints , Servings: 3

Ingredients

- 1 - lb. beef cubes, cut from a chuck roast.
- ¼ - red onion, chopped
- 2 - garlic cloves, crushed
- 1 15 - oz can mushroom, drained
- 2 - cups homemade beef broth
- 2.5 - cups water
- ½ - cup pearled barley
- Salt and pepper to taste
- Fresh parsley to garnish (optional)
- Homemade Bread from the freezer
- 15 - oz. can corn

Instructions:

- Dark-colored the perimeters of the beef 3-D shapes in a good-sized pan with the crimson onion and squashed garlic. When all facets have sautéed, consist of the hamburger inventory and water.
- Heat to the factor of boiling, at that point, include the pearled grain. Let cook at a shifting bubble for 20mints.
- Season with salt and pepper to flavor.
- Get equipped rolls.
- Warm corn as coordinated at the can.
- Serve with bread and corn.

NUTRITION PER SERVING: *Calories: 190 Carbs: 23g Fat: 8g Protein: 9g*

VEGAN WINTER LENTIL STEW

PREP TIME: 10mins COOK TIME: 50mins , SERVINGS: 8

INGREDIENTS

- 2 - Tbsp olive oil
- 1 - yellow onion
- 4 - cloves garlic
- 4 - Carrots (about 1/2 lb.)
- 4 - Stalks celery
- 2 - lbs potatoes
- 1 - cup brown lentils
- 1 - tsp dried rosemary
- ½ - tsp dried thyme
- 2 - Tbsp Dijon mustard
- 1.5 - Tbsp soy sauce
- 1 - Tbsp brown sugar
- 6 - cups vegetable broth
- 1 - cup frozen peas

INSTRUCTIONS
- Bones the onion and mince the garlic. Include the olive oil, onion, and garlic to a huge soup pot and start to sauté over medium warmth.
- While the onion and garlic are sautéing, dice the celery, at that point add it to the pot and keep on sauté. As the celery, onion, and garlic are sautéing, strip and hack the carrots into half adjusts. Add the carrots to the pot and keep on sauté.
- Like the onion, garlic, celery, and carrots are sautéing, strip and 3D square the potatoes into 3/4 to 1-inch pieces. Add the cubed potatoes to the pot alongside the lentils, rosemary, thyme, Dijon, soy sauce, dark colored sugar, and vegetable soup.
- Quickly mix the fixings to join, at that point place a cover on the pot, turn the warmth up to high, and heat the stew up to the point of boiling. When it arrives at a bubble, turn the warmth down to low and give it a chance to stew for 30mints, blending once in a while.
- Close to the part of the bargain, when the potatoes are delicate, start to squash the potatoes a piece as you mix. This will help thicken the stew.

- At last, following 30 minutes, blend in the solidified peas and enable them to warm through. Taste the stew and include salt if necessary (this will rely upon the salt substance of your soup, I didn't include any extra). Serve hot and appreciate!

NUTRITION PER SERVING:
Calories: 213 Carbs: 41g Fat: 5g Protein: 9g

MATZO BALL SOUP

PREP TIME: 10mins COOK TIME: 1hr 30mins, SERVINGS: 5

INGREDIENTS

- **SOUP**
- 1 - Tbsp vegetable
- 2 - cloves garlic
- 1 - yellow onion
- 3 - carrots
- 3 - stalks celery
- 1 - chicken breast
- 6 - cups chicken broth
- 2 - cups of water
- Freshly cracked pepper
- Few sprigs fresh dill
- **MATZO BALLS**
- 3 - large eggs
- 3 - Tbsp vegetable or canola oil
- ¾ - cup matzo meal
- 1 - tsp salt
- ½ - tsp baking powder
- Freshly cracked pepper
- 3 - Tbsp water

INSTRUCTIONS

- Mince the garlic and bones the onion, celery, and carrots. Sauté the garlic, onion, celery, and carrots with the vegetable oil in an enormous pot over medium warmth until the onions are delicate and straightforward.
- Include the chicken bosom, chicken stock, 2 cups water, some crisply split pepper, and a couple of sprigs of dill to the pot. Spot a cover on the pot and let it come up to a bubble. When it arrives at a bubble, turn the warmth down to low and give it a chance to stew for 30mints.
- While the soup is stewing, blend the matzo ball mixture. In a medium bowl, whisk together the eggs and vegetable oil. Include the matzo dinner, salt, heating powder, and a little newly split pepper to the eggs and oil. Blend until all-around joined. At last, include 3 Tbsp water and blend until smooth once more. Refrigerate the blend for 30mints to permit the matzo supper time to retain the dampness.
- After the chicken soup has stewed, cautiously take off the chicken bosom and shred it with a fork. Return the destroyed chicken to the soup. Taste the stock and change the salt if necessary.
- When the matzo ball combination has refrigerated and hardened up, start to frame it into ping pong estimated balls. Drop the balls into the stewing soup as they're fashioned, restoring the top to the pot after everyone. When all of the matzo balls are within the soup, let them stew for 20mints without evacuating the quilt. Ensure the soup is delicately stewing the complete time.
- Include a few sprigs of crisp dill simply earlier than serving.

NUTRITION PER SERVING:
Calories: 120 Carbs: 15g Fat: 5g Protein: 3g

Potato Leek Soup

PREP TIME: 5mins COOK TIME: 25mins , Servings: 6

INGREDIENTS

- 4 - medium leeks, dark green stems removed
- ½ - large white onion, chopped
- 2 - medium russet potatoes, peeled and cut into cubes
- 1 - tablespoon flour, use AP gluten-free flour for GF
- 1 - tbsp butter
- 4 - cups chicken stock, use vegetable broth for vegetarians
- ½ - cup 2% milk
- Salt and fresh pepper

INSTRUCTIONS

- Wash leeks cautiously to expel all coarseness. I normally cut them on a level plane and separate the rings to ensure no soil remains. Coarsely cleave them when washed.
- In a medium soup pot, soften spread and include flour low fire.
- Utilizing a wooden spoon, blend well. This will thicken your soup and give it an awesome flavor.
- Include chicken stock, leeks, onion, potatoes and heat to the point of boiling.
- Spread and stew on low for around 20-25 minutes, until potatoes are delicate.
- Utilizing an inundation blender, mix the soup until smooth including the milk and altering salt and pepper to taste.
- Serve right away.

NUTRITION PER SERVING:
Calories: 133, Carb: 23.5g, Protein: 4.5g, Fat: 2.5g, Sugar: 5g

Chunky Beef, Cabbage, and Tomato Soup

PREP TIME: 10mins COOK TIME: 30mins, Servings: 7

INGREDIENTS
- 1 - lb 90% lean ground beef
- 1 ½ - teaspoon kosher salt
- ½ - cup diced onion
- ½ - cup diced celery
- ½ - cup diced carrot
- 28 - oz can diced or crushed tomatoes
- 5 - cups chopped green cabbage
- 4 - cups beef stock, canned* or homemade
- 2 - bay leaves

INSTRUCTIONS
- INSTANT POT:
- Expecting your electric weight cooker has a saute choice, or if utilizing the Instant Pot, press the saute catch and let the weight cooker gets hot, when hot shower with oil, include the ground hamburger and salt and cook until sautéed separating the meat into little pieces as it cooks, 3 to 4mints.
- Whenever seared, include the onion, celery, and carrots and saute 4 to 5mints.
- Include the tomatoes, cabbage, meat stock, and inlet leaves, lock the cover cook high-weight 20mints.
- Give the steam a chance to discharge normally. Expel cove leaves and serve. Makes 11cups.
- STOVE TOP:
- Pursue indistinguishable headings from above in a huge pot or Dutch stove, cook secured low 40mints.

NUTRITION PER SERVING:
Calories: 181 Carbo: 14g, Protein: 15.5g, Fat: 6g, Sugar: 4.5g.

CHICKEN SOUP WITH SPINACH AND WHOLE WHEAT ACINI DI PEPE

Prep Time: 5mins Cook Time: 25mins, Serves: 4

INGREDIENTS

- 4 - boneless skinless chicken thighs,
- ¼ - teaspoon kosher salt
- 1 - teaspoon olive oil
- ½ - cup diced onion
- ½ - cup diced celery
- ½ - cup peeled and sliced carrot
- 3 - cloves garlic, minced
- 4 - cups low-sodium chicken broth
- 2 - bay leaves
- black pepper, to taste
- 2 - cups baby spinach
- ½ - cup Delallo Whole Wheat Acini di Pepe, 2.5 oz

INSTRUCTIONS

- Season the chicken with salt.
- Warm the oil in a medium nonstick pot over medium warmth. Include the onion, celery, carrot, and garlic and sauté until delicate, 4 to 5mints.
- Include the chicken, stock, inlet leaves, and 1/8 teaspoon dark pepper and heat to the point of boiling. Spread and lessen to medium-low until the chicken shreds effectively, around 25mints.
- Dispose of the cove leaves, coarsely shred the chicken with two forks and come back to the soup, including the pasta and cook as indicated by bundle bearings, including the child spinach at last to wither.

NUTRITION PER SERVING:
Calories: 266, Carb: 25g, Protein: 28g, Fat: 6g, Sugar: 3g.

Cauliflower and Sweet Corn Bisque

Prep Time: 5mins Cook Time: 50mints, Servings: 4

Ingredients:

- 2 to 3 - tablespoons extra-virgin olive oil
- 1 - large onion, chopped
- 1 - small-medium-sized head of cauliflower, chopped
- 2 - cloves garlic, chopped
- 2 - ears sweet corn
- salt to taste

- white pepper to taste
- pinch of cayenne pepper
- 1 - tablespoon butter
- fresh thyme or other fresh herbs for garnish

Instructions:

- Warm the olive oil in a substantial bottomed pot. Include the onions and a spot of salt and cook on low heat, blending once in a while, for 5mints or until translucent.
- Include the hacked cauliflower and garlic and increment warmth to medium. Include another spot of salt alongside white pepper and discretionary cayenne pepper. Cook, blending sometimes until cauliflower is delicately brilliant sautéed and marginally relaxed about 5mints.
- In the meantime, shuck the corn and cut the pieces from both. Put a large portion of the bits in a safe spot, and add the rest of the parts to the pot alongside both of the cobs. Add simply enough water to cover the ears and heat blend to the point of boiling, mixing at times. Diminish to a stew and let cook for 30mints.
- Take off the corn cobs from the soup. Utilizing a hand blender, puree the soup altogether. Add the saved corn parts to the soup and cook a couple of minutes to warm through. Add salt and pepper to taste, and blend in the discretionary spread. Present with the discretionary crisp herbs for trimming.

NUTRITION PER SERVING:_Calories: 200 Carbs: 17g Fat: 13g Protein: 6g_

Cannellini Stewed with Tomatoes and Pancetta

Prep Time: 1hr Cook Time: 30mints , Servings: 6

Ingredients:

- 1 ½ - cups dried cannellini, soaked in at least 3 inches of water to cover overnight
- 2 - tablespoons extra-virgin olive oil
- ¼ - cup – ½ cup finely diced pancetta
- 2 to 3 - cloves garlic, minced
- ½ - cup dry white wine
- 28 - ounce can whole, peeled plum tomatoes
- 2 - cups of water
- Salt and freshly ground black pepper to taste

Instructions:

- Warmth the olive oil in a medium-enormous pot or Dutch broiler over a medium-high fire. Include the pancetta and cook, blending once in a while, until marginally caramelized and firm, around 5-6 minutes.
- Alternatively, blend around a paper towel in the container to retain overabundance oil, and dispose of. Include the garlic and mix an additional 30 seconds or thereabouts. Include the white wine and heat to the point of boiling, mixing to scrape up any cooked bits at the base of the container.
- Channel the doused beans and include the beans, tomatoes and all their juice, and the water. Heat just to the point of boiling, and after that decrease warmth to a low stew.
- Spread and cook at any rate 1 ½hrs, ideally two, until beans are delicate. Season with salt and pepper to taste. Present with a shower of additional olive oil over each bowl.

NUTRITION PER SERVING:
Calories: 101 Carbs: 25g Fat: 1g Protein: 4g

Broccoli Cheese Soup

Prep Time 10mints Cooking Time 30mints, Servings: 8

Ingredients

- ½ - cup butter
- 1 - white onion, diced
- 2 - medium carrots, finely diced
- 2 - stalks of celery, diced very small
- 4 - cups chicken broth
- 2 - heads fresh broccoli, chopped
- 1 - cup milk
- 2 - tablespoons cornstarch
- 1 - teaspoon garlic, minced
- ¼ - teaspoon white pepper
- ¼ - teaspoon dried thyme
- ½ - teaspoon salt
- Dash of nutmeg
- 1 - cup heavy whipping cream
- 12 - ounces white American cheese, cubed

- 16 - ounces sharp cheddar cheese, shredded

Instructions:
- In a big soup pot, include the margarine, onion, carrots, and celery. Cook over medium warmth for around 4 to 5mints until carrots are delicate.
- To the pot, include stock and broccoli. Bubble 10mints to relax the broccoli.
- In a little bowl, include milk, cornstarch, garlic, and all seasonings. Blend well until all cornstarch knots are disintegrated. Empty the cornstarch blend into the soup pot and bring to a low stew.
- Include cheddar and cream. Blend consistently to soften. Mix until cheddar is easily mixed.
- Serve right away.

NUTRITION PER SERVING:
Calories: 150 Carbs: 15g Fat: 7g Protein: 5g

Cream of Asparagus Soup

Prep Time: 5minsTotal Time: 25mins, Servings: 6

INGREDIENTS

- 2 - lbs asparagus, 2 bunches, tough ends snapped off
- 1 - tbsp unsalted butter
- 1 - medium onion, chopped
- 6 - cups reduced-sodium chicken broth
- 2 - tbsp low-fat sour cream
- kosher salt and fresh pepper, to taste

INSTRUCTIONS

- Dissolve margarine over low heat in a huge pot. Include onion and sauté until delicate, around 2mints.
- Cut the asparagus down the middle and add to the pot alongside chicken soup and dark pepper, to taste. Heat to the point of boiling spread and cook low around 20 minutes or until asparagus is exceptionally delicate.
- Take from warmth, include acrid cream and utilizing your handheld blender, puree until smooth.

NUTRITION PER SERVING:

Calories: 81, Carb: 10g, Protein: 6g, Fat: 3, Sugar: 1g,

Gastric Sleeve Dessert Recipes

Stuffed Strawberries

Prep Time: 20mints Total Time: 20, Serving size: 2

Ingredients

- 12 - fresh strawberries
- ⅛ - tsp of vanilla extract
- 4 - Tbsp of fat-free cream cheese softened
- 3 - tsp Stevia
- 1 - low-fat graham cracker crushed into crumbs

Instructions

- Cut the finishes off the strawberries and with a sharp blade cut an X – don't slice through the strawberry. Tenderly expel a little strawberry from the middle.
- In a little bowl blend – cream cheddar, Stevia, and vanilla.
- Spot blend into a baked good pack or a plastic sack with the tip cut off and pipe in the filling.
- Move the top of strawberries in graham wafer scraps.

NUTRITION PER SERVING:
Calories: 34, Fat: 0g, Carb: 8g Protein: 1g Sugars: 2g

Cream Cheese Frosting

Prep Time: 10mins Total Time: 10, Serves: 3

Ingredients

- ½ - cup cream cheese, such as homemade cashew cream cheese
- ½ - tsp pure vanilla extract
- 4 - tbsp powdered sugar
- ¼ - cup silken tofu
- 2 - tbsp milk of choice, as needed for desired thickness

Instructions

- Mix everything together in a little nourishment processor. In case you're utilizing this formula to top cupcakes, I'd prescribe icing them just before serving, or icing prior and afterward putting away the cupcakes in the refrigerator, because of the short-lived nature of the fixings.
- Extra icing can be put away for a couple of days in the cooler, secured. Variety thoughts: Add pumpkin, or destroyed carrot and pineapple for a carrot cake plunge, or cinnamon and pecans.

NUTRITION PER SERVING:
Calories: 20, Fat: 1.5g, Carb: 0.5g Protein: 0.5g Sugar: 0g

Quinoa Sesame Brittle

Prep Time: 10mints Cook Time: 30mints, Servings: 10

Ingredients

- 1 - cup mixed nuts, chopped
- 1/3 - cup uncooked white quinoa
- 1/3 - cup sesame seeds
- 1/8 - teaspoon sea salt
- ½ - cup maple syrup I used medium amber color
- 4 - tablespoons palm sugar
- 2 - tablespoons coconut oil

Instructions

- Preheat stove to 165 degrees C (325 F). Line a heating sheet with material paper. Ensure you spread the whole surface and every one of the edges.
- Consolidate quinoa, blended nuts, sesame seeds, and ocean salt in a major bowl. Blend to join. Put in a safe spot.
- Consolidate coconut oil, maple syrup, and palm sugar in a little pan. Warm over medium-low heat for 2 to 3mints. Blend at times until the oil and maple syrup are all around joined. It's OK that the palm sugar isn't totally broken up now.
- Pour the syrup blend onto the dry fixings. Mix to join and blend all the dry fixings with the fluid.
- Pour everything onto the focal point of the material lined preparing sheet and spread into an even layer with a spatula. Attempt to get it as even as would be prudent. The weak sheet will venture into a more slender layer as it heats.
- Prepare for 15mints. Turn the dish (180 degrees) once to guarantee notwithstanding searing. Prepare for another 15 to 20mints. Watch cautiously during the most recent 5 minutes to forestall consuming. The fragile is done when it's turned out to be profound brilliant dark colored in shading.
- Let cool totally. Break into scaled down pieces with your fingers.
- Store scraps in a fixed pack or holder at room temperature for a multi week, or in the cooler for as long as a multi month.

NUTRITION PER SERVING:
Calories: 151 Carb: 16.9g Protein: 3g Fat: 8.7g Sugar: 8.7g

LEMONADE CUPCAKES

Prep Time 15mins Cook Time 20mins , Servings: 24

Ingredients

- 1 15.25 - oz box of white cake mix
- 1 - cup of water
- 1/3 - cup unsweetened applesauce
- 1 - tbsp lemon zest
- 1 ½ - tbsp sugar-free lemonade mix
- 1 to 8 - oz tub of light whipped topping

Instructions

- Preheat stove to 350. Line 24 biscuit/cupcake cups with paper liners.
- In a medium-sized blending bowl, consolidate cake blend, water, fruit purée, lemon pizzazz and 1 tbsp of the sans sugar lemonade blend.
- Spoon hitter equitably into cupcake cups.
- Prepare until a toothpick embedded into the inside confesses all, about 17mintes. Move cupcakes quickly to a rack to cool.
- While cupcakes are cooling, make the icing by consolidating the whipped fixing, and staying 1/2 tbsp without sugar lemonade blend.
- When cupcakes are totally cool, top with icing and serve.

NUTRITION PER SERVING: *Calories 100 Fat 3g Carb 16.7g Sugars 11.2g Protein 0.8g*

Cherry Chocolate Chip Ice Cream

Prep Time: 20mints Cook Time: 10mints , Servings: 8

INGREDIENTS
- 2 - cups cherries, fresh
- ½ - banana
- ½ - cup unsweetened almond milk
- 3 - tablespoons dairy-free chocolate chips

Instructions:
- Spot all fixings in a microwave-secure mug. Blend with a fork
- Microwave on high for 60seconds
- Appreciate!
- Wash and dry the fruits, and take everything out of the pits. Spot in a cooler percent or glass holder, and stop for at any price three hours. In the occasion which you do not have an opportunity, you may make use of solidified end result.
- Strip a banana, and notice half in the cooler.
- Pour ¼ cup of the almond milk into ice 3-D rectangular plate, and forestall those additionally, for in any occasion three hours.
- Spot the solidified end result, a massive part of a solidified banana, the almond-milk ice 3 - d shapes, and ¼ cup almond milk in a nourishment processor, and manner till definitely easy, a few minutes.
- Blend in chocolate chips, and recognize right away!

NUTRITION PER SERVING:
Calories: 128, Carb: 22.3g, Protein: 2.1g, Fat: 4, Sugar: 17g,

Skinny Mug Brownies

Prep Time 2mins Cook Time 1min Total Time 3mins

Ingredients

- 1 - tablespoon cocoa powder, unsweetened
- 2 - packets Truvia
- 2 - tablespoons all-purpose flour
- 3 - tablespoons almond milk

Instructions

- Spot all fixings in a microwave-safe mug. Blend with a fork or little whisk
- Microwave on high for 60 seconds
- Appreciate!

NUTRITION PER SERVING:

Calories: 97 Carbs: 9g Fat: 2g Protein: 1g

Chocolate Peanut Butter Microwave Cake

PREP TIME: 1min COOK TIME: 1min , Serving: 1

INGREDIENTS
- 2 - tablespoons powdered peanut butter
- 1 - tablespoon unsweetened cocoa powder
- 1 - tablespoon all-purpose flour
- 1 - tablespoon packed brown sugar
- 1 - teaspoon baking powder
- 3 - tablespoons liquid egg whites
- 1 - tablespoon water

INSTRUCTIONS
- Whisk together all fixings in a little blending bowl until all around joined. Move to a microwave-safe ramekin, mug or bowl.
- Microwave at 70% for 40 seconds, or until the cake is cooked to your ideal gooeyness. Keep in mind, microwave power levels drastically.
- The first run through making a microwave cake, keep a nearby eye as to not over-cook the cake.

NUTRITION PER SERVING:
Calories: 130 Carbs: 3 Fat: 7g Protein: 14g

Triple Berry Cobbler

Prep: 15mins Slow-Cook: 3hrs (low) + 1 hour (high) Cool: 30mins
Servings: 12

Ingredients
- Nonstick cooking spray
- 1 14 - ounce package frozen loose-pack mixed berries
- 1 21 - ounce can blueberry pie filling
- 2 - tablespoons sugar
- 1 6.5 - ounce package blueberry muffin mix
- ⅓ - cup water
- 2 - tablespoons vegetable oil
- Plain Greek yogurt (optional)
- Honey (optional)

Instructions:
- Daintily coat a 3 ½ or 4 ½ moderate cooker with a cooking splash; put in a safe spot.
- In cooker consolidate solidified berries, pie filling, and sugar.
- Spread and cook on low-heat setting for 3 hours. Go cooker to a high-warm setting. In a medium bowl consolidate biscuit blend, the water, and oil; mix just until joined. Spoon biscuit blend over berry blend.
- Spread and cook for 1 hour more or until a wooden toothpick embedded into the focal point of biscuit blend tells the truth. Mood killer cooker. In the event that conceivable, expel earthenware liner from cooker. Cool, revealed, for 30 to 45mints on a wire rack before serving.
- Whenever wanted, present with yogurt and nectar.

NUTRITION PER SERVING:
Calories 162, Fat 2, Sugar 14g, 1g protein

Dark Chocolate Mint Bites

Prep: 30mins Chill: 15mins + 1hr, SERVERS: 8

Ingredients

- Nonstick cooking spray
- 1 - cup quick-cooking rolled oats
- ¾ - cup dark or semisweet chocolate pieces
- ¼ - cup unsalted butter
- 1 - cup finely crushed chocolate wafers
- 1 - tablespoon unsweetened cocoa powder
- ¼ - teaspoon salt
- 1 - teaspoon shortening
- 1 - cup powdered sugar
- 2 - tablespoons reduced-fat cream cheese, softened
- 1 - tablespoon low-fat milk
- ½ - teaspoon peppermint extract
- ½ - teaspoon vanilla
- 1 - drop green food coloring (optional)

Instructions:

- Line an 8x8x2-inch heating container with foil, expanding foil over the edges of the dish. Coat foil with cooking splash. Put in a safe spot.
- For the outside layer, in nourishment processor beat oats until fine. In a medium, pan consolidates 1/4 cup of the chocolate pieces and the spread; warmth and mix until liquefied. Blend in the handled oats, finely squashed chocolate wafers, cocoa powder, and salt. Press hull blend into the base of the readied dish. Chill for 15mints.
- In a similar pot consolidate the remaining ½ cup chocolate pieces and the shortening. Warmth and mix over low heat until liquefied and smooth. Put in a safe spot.
- In a medium bowl join powdered sugar, cream cheddar, milk, peppermint concentrate, vanilla, and, whenever wanted, sustenance shading; mix until smooth. Spread over outside. Shower with the liquefied chocolate blend.
- Chill around 1 hour or until set. Utilizing the edges of the foil, lift the whole bars out of the container. Cut into 24 bars.

NUTRITION PER SERVING:
Calories 105, Fat 1g, Carb, 1g, sugar 9g, Protein 1g.

Butterscotch Bars

Prep Time: 10mints Cook Time: 30 mints , Servings: 15

Ingredients

- 1 - cup packed brown sugar
- 5 - tablespoons butter, melted
- 1 - teaspoon vanilla extract
- 1 - large egg, lightly beaten
- 9 - ounces all-purpose flour
- 2 ½ - cups quick-cooking oats
- ½ teaspoon salt
- ½ - teaspoon baking soda Cooking spray
- ¾ - cup fat-free sweetened condensed milk
- 1 ¼ cups butterscotch morsels
- 1/8 - teaspoon salt
- ½ - cup finely chopped walnuts, toasted

Instructions:

- Preheat stove to 350°.
- Consolidate sugar and spread in an enormous bowl. Mix in vanilla and egg. Gauge or delicately spoon flour into dry estimating cups; level with a blade. Join flour, oats, ½ teaspoon salt, and preparing the soft drink in a bowl.
- Add oat blend to sugar blend; mix with a fork until consolidated. Spot 3 cups oat blend into the base of a 13 x 9-inch heating dish covered with a cooking splash; press into the base of the skillet. Put in a safe spot.
- Spot improved consolidated milk, butterscotch pieces, and 1/8 teaspoon salt in a microwave-safe bowl; microwave at HIGH 1 moment or until butterscotch pieces dissolve, blending at regular intervals. Blend in pecans.
- Scratch blend into the dish, spreading equitably over outside. Sprinkle equally with residual oat blend, tenderly squeezing into the butterscotch blend. Heat at 350° for 30mints. Spot skillet on a cooling rack; run a blade around outside edge. Cool totally.

NUTRITION PER SERVING:
Calories 148 Fat 5.1g Carb 23.4g

Gastric Sleeve Smoothie Recipes

Frozen Peach Bellini Mocktail

Time: 5mins, Servings: 2

Ingredients
- 2 - ripe peaches, peeled and sliced
- 1 - cup sparkling apple juice, plus more for serving
- 2 - teaspoons SPLENDA Sugar Blend
- 1 - teaspoon lime juice

Instructions
- Spot cut peaches in the cooler for 60mints.
- Join peaches, 1 cup shimmering squeezed apple, Sugar Blend, and lime squeeze in a blender and mix until smooth.
- Fill 2 glasses and include around 1/2 inch of extra shining squeezed apple.

NUTRITION PER SERVING:
Calories: 138 Carbs: 31g Fat: 0g Protein: 2g

Mixed Melon Cucumber Coolers

Prep Time 10mins, Servings: 2

Ingredients

- 2 - cups cubed seedless watermelon
- 1 ½ - cups cubed cantaloupe
- 3 - inch piece of cucumber, peeled and cut into chunks, plus extra slices for garnish
- ½ - ounce fresh lime juice
- Club soda

Instructions

- Join watermelon, melon, cucumber and lime squeeze in a blender and heartbeat until a thick squeeze structures.
- Fill two glasses with ice and gap the juice equally among the two glasses.
- Top each glass with shining water and slide a couple of additional cucumber cuts down within the glass for included flavor. Appreciate!

NUTRITION PER SERVING:

Calories: 120 Carbs: 28g Fat: 0g Protein: 2g

Healthy Pink Drink Strawberry Refresher

Prep Time 5mints Total Time 5mints, Servings: 1

Ingredients

- 1 - cup unsweetened strawberry sparkling water like bubbly
- ¼ - cup freeze-dried strawberries
- ½ - cup coconut milk from carton

Instructions

- Pour solidify dried strawberries in a serving cup at that point pour Perrier strawberry shining water over. Mix well and let sit for two or three minutes to soak. Add ice to glass at that point pour coconut milk over. Blend and serve.

NUTRITION PER SERVING:
Calories 313, Fat 7g Carb 56g Sugar 40g

Raspberry and Fig Hibiscus Cooler

Prep Time 10mints Total Time 20mints , Serves 2

INGREDIENTS
- 3 - tablespoons dried hibiscus flowers
- 2 - tablespoons raw honey
- ½ - cup fresh raspberries
- 2 - ripe figs
- 3 - sprigs mint plus extra to garnish
- lime wedges

Instructions:
- Set the hibiscus blooms in a box and spread with 1/2cups of bubbling water. Let soak for 5mints. Strain the tea into every other box, eliminating the blooms. Include the nectar and mix till disintegrated.
- Place the tea in the Fridge even as you set up the remainder of the beverage. In another container or a combined drink shaker jumble the raspberries, figs, and mint till all-around beaten and fragrant.
- Include the cooled tea, mix it nicely, and press the blend to dispose of the mash. Share the tea equally among two glasses. Top it with ice a lime wedge and a sprig of mint.

NUTRITION PER SERVING:
Calories: 110 Carbs: 20g Fat: 3g Protein: 1g

Non-Alcoholic Ginger Mimosa

Prep time: 3mins Total time: 3mins, Servings: 4

INGREDIENTS
- ½ - Fresh Orange Juice, Chilled
- 1 –Tsp Maple Syrup
- 16 – Oz Ginger Ale
- 4 – Pieces, Fresh Ginger, Sliced Into 1 Inch
- 1 - Oranges, Sliced
- Ice Cubes

INSTRUCTIONS:
- Take a pitcher, include squeezed orange, maple syrup and blend well.
- Presently include ice blocks and shake well once more.
- Include soda and mix well.
- Fill two tall glasses with the readied non-alcoholic ginger mimosa.
- Top with orange cuts, ginger cuts and serve.

NUTRITION PER SERVING:
Calories: 150 Carbs: 38g Fat: 0g Protein: 1g

Mango Meyer Lemon Margarita Mocktails

Prep time: 10mins Total time: 10mins, Servings: 4

Ingredients

- 6 - tablespoons fresh mango puree
- 3 to 4 - tablespoons simple syrup
- 2 - tablespoons fresh Meyer lemon juice
- 16 - oz (500 ml) sparkling water
- **For sugaring the rims of the glasses:**
- 1 - Meyer lemon wedge
- Coarse sugar
- Other:
- Ice cubes
- Fresh sprigs of mint, for garnish

Instructions

- Whisk together the mango puree, straightforward syrup, and lemon squeeze in an enormous pitcher. Quickly blend in the water, being mindful so as not to over-mix and lose all the carbonation.
- To sugar, the edges of the glasses, rub a lemon wedge along the edge of each glass and after that plunge it into coarse sugar.
- Put a couple of ice 3D shapes in each glass, pour in the beverage, and top each with a mint sprig.
- Serve right away.

NUTRITION PER SERVING:
Calories: 170 Carbs: 26g Fat: 0g Protein: 0g

RASPBERRY PEACH LEMONADE

Prep Time: 15mins , Servings: 8

INGREDIENTS

- **RASPBERRY PEACH PUREE:**
- 4 - fresh peaches, pitted, diced into large chunks
- 1 - cup fresh raspberries
- 1 ¼ - cups water

SIMPLE SYRUP:

- ½ - cup granulated sugar
- ½ - cup water

LEMONADE:

- 7 - cups cold water
- 1 ¼ - cups fresh lemon juice
- ice cubes
- Extra raspberries, for garnish optional
- Extra peach slices, for garnish optional
- mint sprigs, for garnish optional

INSTRUCTIONS

- Include diced peaches, raspberries and water to a sustenance processor or blender and procedure until pureed.
- Spot a strainer over a huge blending bowl and empty the peach raspberry puree into the sifter. Utilize the back of a huge spoon to drive the puree around so the fluid falls through the sifter and seeds/skin remain inside the strainer.
- Dispose of seeds/skin from the sifter and set blending bowl with fluid in it aside.
- Include granulated sugar and 1/2 cup water to a little pan and warmth over MED heat until sugar disintegrates into the water, blending sometimes. The bubble around 3 minutes until the fluid has turned out to be syrupy. Put aside to cool somewhat.
- Include 7 cups water, lemon squeeze, and ice blocks to a huge pitcher. Blend to join. Pour in cooled straightforward syrup and peach raspberry fluid. Mix to consolidate once more.
- Store shrouded in the fridge until prepared to serve. Serve chilled with enhancements, whenever wanted

NUTRITION PER SERVING:

Calories: 150 Carbs: 39g Fat: 0g Protein: 0g

RAINBOW COCONUT WATER SPRITZERS

Prep Time 5mins Total time: 15 MINS, SERVES: 4

INGREDIENTS

- **HANDFULS OF FRESH:**

- raspberries
- strawberries
- cherries
- peaches
- pineapple
- lime slices
- fresh mint
- blueberries
- blackberries
- 16 - ounces coconut water
- 8 - ounces flavored seltzer such as coconut e.t.c

INSTRUCTIONS

- Fill each glass with a touch of squashed ice, at that point include the natural product in rainbow hues. I like utilizing the ROY G BIV rules! When the organic product is in the glasses, include more ice and fill each glass with around 4 ounces of coconut water.
- Finish each off with some seasoned seltzer and serve. Enhancement with extra crisp mint.

NUTRITION PER SERVING:*Calories: 140 Carbs: 22g Fat: 7g Protein: 1g*

PINEAPPLE PEACH AGUA FRESCA

Prep Time 10mins Total time: 30mins, SERVES: 4

INGREDIENTS

- 3 - ripe peaches, peeled and cubed
- 1 - cup fresh pineapple chunks
- 2 - cups of water
- 3 - limes, juiced
- 2 - tablespoons simple syrup
- 1 - cup frozen peach slices
- fresh mint
- lime slices for serving

INSTRUCTIONS

- To make the straightforward syrup, join equivalent amounts of sugar and water, in a pan over medium warmth. rush until the sugar breaks down and stew for a moment or two, at that point expel from the warmth and let cool totally.
- Include the peaches, pineapple and 1 cup of water to a blender and mix until totally pureed. Utilizing a fine-work sifter, empty the puree through into an enormous bowl or estimating cup, utilizing a spoon to press the remainder of the fluid out when you get as far as possible.
- Consolidate the juice with the rest of the water, lime juice and straightforward syrup in a huge pitcher. Taste and include more syrup whenever wanted.
- Chill until virus. Prior to serving, include the solidified peach cuts alongside a couple of ice 3D squares in the event that you'd like it very cold.
- Serve over squashed ice the additional lime cuts and mint.

NUTRITION PER SERVING:
Calories: 121 Carbs: 32g Fat: 0g Protein: 1g

Conclusion

Sleeve gastrectomy is a profitable weapon in the battle against metabolic disorder and weight. Abundance weight reduction, goals of diabetes, hypertension, rest apnoea and cardiovascular renovating with a decrease in heart hazard profile, give convincing contentions to the extension of metabolic medical procedure. The biomedical research potential from particular anatomical changes in the gut, happening in a controlled way during medical procedure, is motivating. The coordinated effort among careful and research facility groups reveals new insight into the pathogenesis of metabolic disorder and diabetes, through the adequacy of gastrointestinal medical procedure, and envoys in another time prodded by the need to check the plague.

CPSIA information can be obtained
at www.ICGtesting.com
Printed in the USA
LVHW062125130522
718697LV00005B/124

9 781804 341421